ENDORSEME

"The Man's Guide to Infertility is an informative and easy-to-read guide, written with sensitivity and care. After I took care of Jon and treated his male infertility, he and his partner Laura felt they wanted to help other men navigate the truly difficult journey, which is male infertility. Laura and Jon's efforts have culminated in this clear and comprehensive book.

It delivers an overview of the important topics; explaining the physical, emotional and relationship pressures that people may experience when trying to conceive. Jon and Laura have combined medical insight from leading doctors, compassionate advice, and stories of their own difficult journey to parenthood in a unique way that helps the reader understand the obstacles men may face when trying to build a family with the key steps to overcoming them.

I'm looking forward to recommending it to my patients."

— *Dr Darren Katz, Urologist and Male Fertility Microsurgeon, Medical Director of Men's Health Melbourne, www.menshealthmelbourne.com.au*

"This is a warm, humorous, heartfelt look into the world of IVF, specifically the male experience of infertility. Laura and Jon share their story, their wisdom, and lessons learned with compassion, leaving the reader crying and laughing along the journey."

— *Dr Lora Shahine, MD, reproductive endocrinologist at Pacific NW, Fertility in Seattle, WA, best selling author of 'Not Broken: An Approachable Guide to Miscarriage and Recurrent Pregnancy Loss' and host of Baby or Bust podcast www.drlorashahine.com*

"Jon and Laura were always determined to have a baby. They faced their infertility head on and leaned on each other when times were tough. Despite what they were going through, they both kept raising awareness about male infertility and I'm sure they made a difference to many people's lives. IVF is such an emotional journey, but when I see a happy ending like Jon and Laura had, it truly confirms that I have the best job in the world. "

— *Dr Lynn Burmeister, Medical Director and founder of No.1 Fertility, Fertility Specialist, Obstetrician & Gynaecologist (MBBS FRANZCOG CREI) www.number1fertility.com*

"Finally, a resource that covers the ENTIRE experience of infertility. This book embraces the human side of what can be the most challenging thing many of us ever experience. It is real, comprehensive and relatable, and perfectly covers aspects of the fertility journey that are often considered too difficult or awkward to talk about. "

— *Dr Scott Shemer, Obstetrician and IVF Dad, https://drscottshemer.com.au*

"As someone whose husband is infertile, *The Man's Guide to Infertility* beautifully balances the sensitivities and triggers of infertility with a lighthearted touch. Plus, invaluable insight and advice. We love this book! "

— *Eloise Edington CEO / Founder, The Ribbon Box, www.theribbonbox.com*

"Finally! A resource to help men navigate the challenging journey of infertility and give a voice to their experiences.

This guide is so needed for men and their partners wanting to grow their families. The conversation about infertility is often focused on women's experiences, and it's about time that men had support and resources as well.

I wish we had a resource like this to support my partner when we were going through infertility treatment."

— *Sarah Jefford, Family Creation Lawyer, https://sarahjefford.com*

"What an amazing resource Jon and Laura have created here! Researched and fact-based with personal and moving commentary throughout. A fertility journey can be complex to navigate both in terms of emotions and medical treatments, yet this guide explains everything in terms that are easy to understand and backed by illustrated examples and information from medical professionals. In short, it's a great and informative read which everybody - no matter at which stage of their fertility journey they may be - will benefit from reading"

— *Morten G. Ulsted, CEO & Co-Founder, ExSeed Health,*
  Home Sperm Testing and Fertility Support, www.exseedhealth.com

"A powerful and practical guide to infertility. This book has been needed for a while and I'm glad it's finally out there! Fertility treatment can really take a mental toll on men, this book will help those going through it realise they're not alone."

— *Chris Lawson, IVFDad, www.ivfdad.com*

"What Jon and Laura have put together here is nothing short of remarkable. Providing easily digestible information for what is a complex and emotive subject isn't easy, but they've done it. They have entwined expert knowledge with their lived experience, all whilst helping break down the stigma of male infertility. This book is essential reading for any man navigating the pain of fertility struggles. It is a literary arm around the shoulder, providing the reassurance that you are not alone."

— *Shaun Greenaway, aka @knackered_knackers*

"This book takes all the complexities of infertility and lays it out in an entertaining, fun and digestible way. Jon and Laura have a special way of communicating all facets of the infertility journey like no one else. In the past, infertility education has been designed towards females only. It is so refreshing to finally see material that was designed for and by a man who gets it. This book is a breakthrough within the fertility community, giving men the chance to truly be part of this experience. This is the book to help you get there, with a little chuckle along the way."

— *Emily Getz, Founder of Day 1 Fertility, www.day1fertility.com*

"A great, informative read and every guy should take a look."

— *Toby Trice, British racing driver raising awareness for fertility through motorsport.*
  https://tobytriceracing.com

"Jon and Laura have approached the difficult topic of infertility with a wealth of understanding and empathy; providing a great mix of professional information, personal insights, and useful tools to help you on your fertility journey. A wonderful resource for any man struggling with infertility."

— *Tasha Jennings, Fertility Naturopath, @tashajenningsnd, https://tashajennings.com.au/checklistinfertilityman*

"I loved this book! As a man who went through infertility, I felt so alone and out of the loop. Men need as much support through this process as women do, and this book does an amazing job with support, knowledge, and awareness."

— *Eli Weinstein, Licensed Clinical Social Work Therapist, Host of The Dude Therapist Podcast, www.eliweinsteinlcsw.com*

"This is an incredible book, honest and thoughtful, a must-have for anyone facing the reality of infertility. Jon and Laura have produced a master class with this book, it's truly amazing."

— *Ciaran Hannington, Base Camp for Fertility 2022 and founder of Humanity Health and Fitness*

"A great encyclopaedia for guys going through fertility treatment, the perfect mix of facts and humour touch the mind and soul."

— *Tony Suckling, The Hopeful Father, @ thehopefulfather*

"This is such an amazing book. It has been needed for so long! Wherever you are on your fertility journey, this book will give you the knowledge to get you where you want to be."

— *Kevin Button, founder of The Man Cave, @them_ancave*

"I recommend this book for those looking for a step-by-step, first person account of what it's like for an infertile man trying to conceive. Great details, insights, and drawings that personalize the experience in a fun, personal account."

— *Eric Schwartzman, Dad to Donor Conceived Kids, @ life_di_dad*

"Infertility is something that no one can truly understand unless they've experienced it themselves. People try to but often they just don't get it, but this book helps drastically in that regard. It is the complete guide to infertility, taking into account every perspective and every step of the long trek towards hopefully welcoming a baby.

Traditionally, infertility has been looked at as a woman's issue, but that is a misguided and outdated myth and this book reaffirms that notion.

It wonderfully tackles all aspects of the infertility minefield, including the physical, emotional, financial and psychological side of the often lonely and frustrating journey.

An absolute must-read for any couple or person struggling to conceive, or anyone interested in the subject. A brilliant resource for all, lovingly told by Jon and Laura."

— *Nick Smart, Sports Reporter, Herald Sun*

THE MAN'S GUIDE TO
INFERTILITY

JON & LAURA SUMMERS

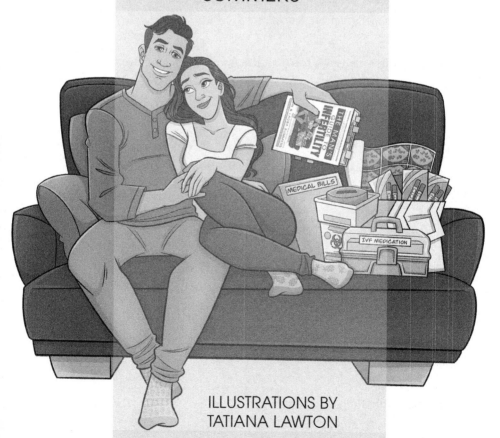

ILLUSTRATIONS BY
TATIANA LAWTON

Summers, Jon & Laura (authors)
THE MAN'S GUIDE TO INFERTILITY
ISBN 978-0-6456050-2-0 (paperback)
Fertility & Infertility - Men's Health

Published by Tall Story Publishing
Typeset Eigerdals 9/16
Book Illustrations by Tatiana Lawton
Photo by Seeds Photography

DEDICATION

For Laura

Our eyes met, and you took my breath away.

The rest is history, miracles really do happen.

For Jon

Everything is possible with you.

CONTENTS

CONTENTS

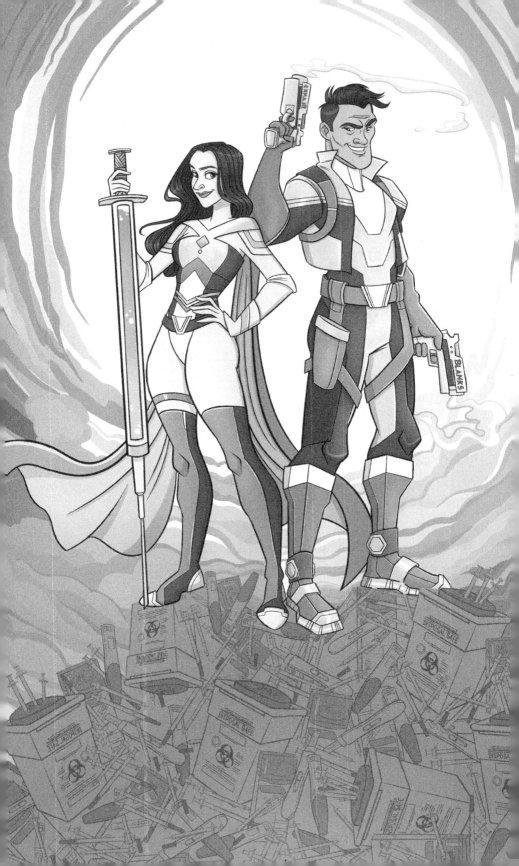

BEING INFERTILE IS LIKE JOINING THE WORST CLUB IN THE WORLD, BUT A CLUB WITH THE BEST MEMBERS.

WELCOME TO THE CLUB!

Before we start, we'd love to give you some useful information to help you as you navigate infertility.

Visit the special page on our website for readers of *The Man's Guide to Infertility*: **www.InfertilityMan.com/MansGuide**

- ▶ Download lists and useful printouts that will help as you are experiencing infertility, including a Fertility Calendar, IVF Budget Template and a list of questions to ask your doctor.

- ▶ See funny videos showing the authors through years of infertility.

- ▶ Download IVF Milestone Cards to use through your own fertility treatment.

- ▶ See the cartoons in the book in full colour.

- ▶ Join The Men's Infertility Group to connect with other men who are going through similar experiences.

DISCLAIMER

We believe everyone has the right to have a family, regardless of gender, sexual orientation or relationship status. This book is intended for men experiencing infertility in some form or another. While we acknowledge and honour the fact that there are many situations where people experience infertility and bring children into their families, this book includes the topic of conception, which requires male and female oocytes and an oven to cook your bun in.

There are many books targeting women trying to get pregnant, but not a lot for men. Our intention is never to exclude anyone, only to focus on a group that had largely been ignored before now. We encourage you to take from this book any information that helps you and then move forward to share ideas and advice with people who have experiences similar to your own. We hope you will find value in this information and adapt it to your personal situation.

The authors' personal experience lies with heterosexual infertility, so this information is based on that learned knowledge. For this book, we will use the pronouns 'he' and 'she'. We acknowledge these words do not include everyone. We hope you will take and apply the information that is relevant to you. If you are a single person seeking fertility treatment, we hope that this information will be of benefit to you as well.

We should say upfront that we're not medical experts in fertility, although Jon does work in healthcare as a paramedic. You must seek medical advice that is tailored to your own circumstances before making decisions. In fact, we have kept the information as free from medical jargon as possible. If there is a word that you would like to clarify, there is a glossary at the end of this book.

Best practice in fertility treatment is constantly changing, with improvements being developed all the time. You will need to speak to professionals who can give you the most up-to-date care. We want to talk you through the basics of fertility treatment but go more in depth about the emotional and social aspects of being infertile. The only way you'll have the stamina to make it through the rigours of fertility treatment is if you have good support systems and a handle on the challenges ahead.

We're so grateful to the people who have shared their fertility stories with us for this book. Names have been changed to protect their privacy.

INTRODUCTION

If you are reading this book, you have decided that at some point in your adult life, you would like help to conceive a child or have a family. Maybe it is something that you have wanted since you were young, or maybe it is a new goal. You might be hoping to build a family with your partner or maybe you have decided to have a child on your own. Perhaps you are supporting a friend to conceive a child. Or maybe you are donating sperm for another family. There are so many reasons that men come to fertility treatment.

Maybe you already have a diagnosis and you know you can't conceive without medical intervention. Perhaps you had a fun conversation where you and your partner decided 'This is it. It's time!' You threw away the condoms, and she went off the pill. You expected you would conceive quickly, and you waited excitedly, expecting to be pregnant in a matter of months.

You waited …
and waited …
and waited …

For many men, a fertility diagnosis brings emotional turmoil, including feelings of guilt, fear and concern. Men can get stuck at the point of diagnosis, not knowing what to do next. They can feel invisible on their fertility journey as doctors and nurses tend to focus more attention on women. The idea of using donor sperm can take an incredible emotional toll, as men feel this is the one thing they should be able to provide. Many men feel negative emotions as they watch their partners suffer, both with the burden of fertility treatment and also the pain that they may feel for their missing baby.

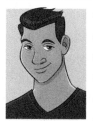 *Many people need to hear these stories and the partners' stories are rarely told. A lot of focus is on the Mums, but not a lot on the Dads or the second Mums or whatever the situation is – they are not often talked about. And we can find it pretty tough too, particularly because our most cherished loved one is going through absolute hell. Almost always we have no control and very little ability to help them and that can be traumatic too. I don't think that is spoken about enough. - Daniel*

Since you're here reading this book, it seems like you might have a bit of a challenge in front of you. You want to conceive a child or become a dad but it turns out that it is not as easy as they made it seem in sex education class.

What if you can't make babies the regular way? What if you and your partner can't conceive naturally? How do you manage your life while undergoing fertility treatment? How do you take care of your relationship when you are both under extra pressure? How do you deal with these challenges while maintaining your mental health?

There is a way.

You can grow through this experience while providing support, care, and resources to your loved ones as you navigate the world of infertility.

This book is your guide through that world.

Each man reading this book will come from different situations. Perhaps you have a wife or a girlfriend. Maybe you're in a same-sex relationship. Perhaps you're stepping up to be a sperm donor for someone you care about. However you got here, you're here because you want to conceive a child (or several of them) or create a family in another way.

Most resources about infertility are focused on women. There are lots of books, websites, influencers, social media groups, films and resources that speak to women about infertility. Not much is aimed at men, which is weird, because half of infertility issues are due to the sperm part of the equation, otherwise known as male factor infertility. Men may supply the sperm or they may support their partner as she goes through fertility treatments ... so where are the guides for men? Men should have support and information to help them through this challenging journey.

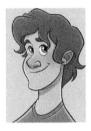

*I felt helpless. No one was talking about this stuff. You'd go online and there was no male conversation. I'd Google 'problems having a baby' or 'fertility issues', and the websites that came up were all pink. I'd post in a forum and women would respond on behalf of their husbands. There was nothing for men. ~ **Matt***

Maybe your wife, girlfriend, partner, or female counterpart handed this book to you. You may have had some assistance in coming to this information. It doesn't matter how you got here or why you are experiencing infertility. You are so much more than 'the guy who provides the sperm'.

In our current climate of instant gratification, comfort and ease, you have been thrown a curve ball: infertility. If you hide from this challenge, disengage, disconnect, leave it all up to your partner, step back and wimp out, then everyone suffers. The good news is if you can rise up and take on this challenge with love, strength and compassion, then you will become an even better version of yourself.

Infertility can bring you to your knees and tear relationships apart. Or it can be a journey of self-discovery that gives your life and your relationships true meaning and purpose. It can be the key that unlocks your heart and brings you closer together. Overcoming infertility can unleash the most vulnerable and authentic version of you. This is your opportunity to step up as a partner and as a father, even before you have kids.

Our most important piece of advice is this: ask for help. Whether you are just starting out on your infertility journey and need some advice or you've been at this for a while and you want to connect with others who have been through it, contact us, message us, get in touch via our website. Make sure you sign up for our support group, our email newsletter, and follow us on social media. We would love to be there for you, not just through the pages of this book. There are so many people out there who are going through a similar experience, you are not alone.

www.InfertilityMan.com

MEET JON & LAURA

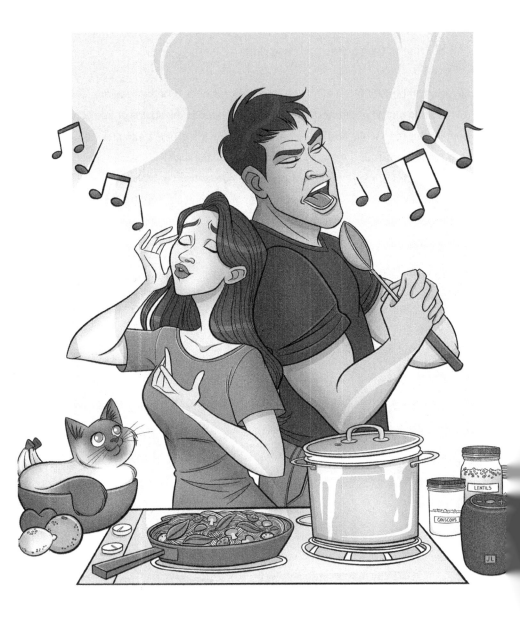

FROM JON

'One nut is better than no nut.'

So we can get off on the right foot, let me introduce myself...

To be honest, I don't blame you for looking at your infertility situation and wanting to run for the hills. This is some heavy stuff. I never expected that I would be someone who would write a book about infertility.

I played rugby, partied a lot and trashed my body throughout my twenties, and then I was a bodybuilder and ran triathlons in my thirties. I had testicular cancer and lost one of my nuts in the surgery that saved my life. I found out that my sperm count was zero, did IVF and had some intense sperm seeking surgeries and now I'm a Dad. I have lived through infertility and I made it to the other side, and so will you.

Infertility is a really difficult experience, and it can come as a huge shock. It is an enormous challenge that affects every area of your life. The most important thing I can share with you is that you are not alone. So many people experience infertility and there is support available to help you through. At the very least, I would love to be a support to you, so feel free to reach out to me online. This book is our contribution to a community that stood by us through our toughest days; we wrote it to pay it forward.

I'm writing this book with my partner and she's an IVF warrior too. She went through 17 pelvic surgeries, thousands of injections, hundreds of blood tests, many pelvic exams and loads of crazy mood-altering hormone drugs for three years before finally giving birth to our kids.

We shared our infertility story online through videos and photos.
You can watch at www.infertilityman.com/videos

We're going to explain some of what happens to you when you're receiving
treatment for infertility, so you're not freaked out by all this new stuff. Then
we're going to share some ideas on how to get it handled and how to do
it with strength and sensitivity. In the end, you don't need to understand
all the medical details, but you do need to know how to deal with medical
professionals, how to take care of yourself through this difficult time, how to
be an understanding and supportive partner, and perhaps how to be the guy
who can add some humour and kindness to lighten the mood. We'll also give
you some tips on how to give a sperm sample, because you'll need to know
how to do that too.

I guarantee that if you apply the information in this book to your own life,
your relationships, and your fertility, you will find it to be a game changer.
If you can support yourself and your partner (or baby-making team) through
infertility with love, strength and humour, then you will become a force to be
reckoned with.

FROM LAURA

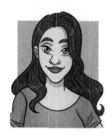

We took a long time to find each other. Both of us spent our early adult life working in jobs we loved, travelling the world and falling in love (but never with the right person). We both always wanted to have children and would probably have liked to have them sooner, but life didn't work out that way.

Jon and I met at a conference. He was 41 and I was 35. We had an instant connection. When we met, it wasn't like meeting someone; it was more like recognising someone. We had spent so much time looking for each other that the moment we saw each other, it was almost obvious.

I was nearing the age where I was starting to wonder if I had missed my chance to have children. I never intended to do that (I think this is the case for many women). When I met Jon, everything suddenly made sense. He was the one I had been looking for all along.

We went on our first date, and it was lovely. We talked, and I felt like I had known him for years. I'm not sure whether he did this on all his first dates, but he mentioned he had previously had testicular cancer and had been told that he couldn't have kids. I'm not sure what I thought this meant at the time. Somehow my brain didn't quite make the connection that this would make it impossible to have children naturally. I don't even really remember how I responded, except that Jon has since told me that I questioned him:

"Is that really true? Have you had it tested recently?"

That was the start of our fertility journey... on our very first date.

Testing Jon's fertility began at the very start of our relationship. Initially, I just left it up to Jon and put the conversation in the back of my mind. He took himself to the doctors and saw a fertility specialist. Brochures and flyers with giant sperm on them quietly showed up at the house.

We knew from the start that we could never conceive naturally.

For us, it was a big jump straight to IVF.

More than anything, this experience teaches you how strong you really are. I thought I was tough before, but through IVF treatment I found untapped reserves of resilience I never knew I had. I have met people with extraordinary infertility challenges who are able to find the strength to keep going despite incredible sadness and crushing disappointments.

The one thing we always believed is that if we kept doing 'the next right thing', then one day infertility would end for us. And it always ends, in one way or another. After an incredibly challenging process, if you just keep taking the next step, and then the next one, and then the next one, eventually you will find a way to be parents or you will make peace with your situation. Somehow, it helped me to know that even if it didn't end the way we wanted it to, this time in our lives couldn't last forever.

Hopefully, we all come out the other side as more resilient and more compassionate people.

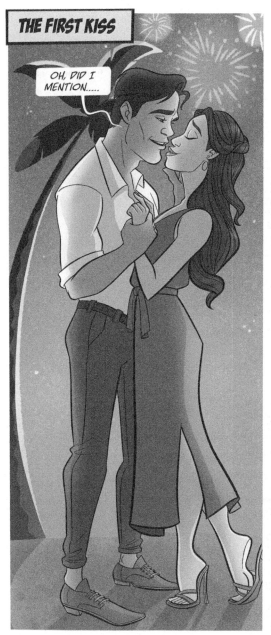

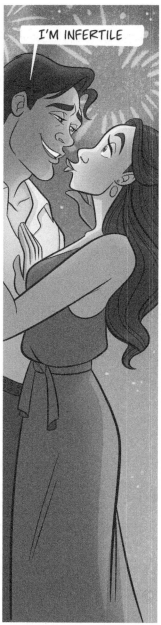

ARE YOU IN THIS OR NOT?

The challenge of infertility is in front of you. This is the point when you need to make a decision.

We have spent enough time in fertility clinic waiting rooms to understand that it is typically the woman who drives this fertility thing. For whatever reason, it tends to be the women, either through nurture or nature, who are more driven to want to have a baby. When there are challenges, the women are usually the ones to first pursue fertility treatment.

We have sat in enough fertility clinic waiting rooms to see that some men can be a bit passive and disengaged. Many do not attend the doctor's appointments and if they do, they aren't really present. Some guys leave it all up to their partner. They step back because it is all a bit too hard.

And some men are amazing. They are there every step of the way, holding their partner's hand, administering the injections and picking her up from the hospital. They are right there to support, taking care of the housework, cooking dinner and doing the washing. They are earning money to pay for fertility treatment and medications, they are managing the paperwork and paying the doctor's invoices. They are the shoulder to cry on, the arms to hold her and the smile that celebrates when things go well.

They are committed.

This journey is challenging. Even if you aren't the partner who has to do the bulk of the medical procedures, the egg retrievals, the transfers and hopefully carry the baby, you are an important member of the team. You just need to be a little more proactive in figuring out the best way to help and be involved.

So, decide. Are you in this or not?

The choice to have children or not can be a deal breaker in relationships. If you don't want to have children and your partner does, then you need to make some difficult choices about your future together.

If it is something you really want, then you need to be an active, contributing and enthusiastic participant in creating your family. Just as you will be if or when you become a father. As most fertility treatment focuses on the partner with the ovaries and the uterus, the other partner needs to work a little harder to figure out how they can contribute, but it is possible.

The choice is yours.

As soon as you choose to be in this, you need to be all in.

If you choose to accept the challenge, you will grow as a man, you will grow in your relationship, and you will grow in your empathy and understanding of the world around you.

If you are fully and totally in, it's time to push the button and commit 100 percent.

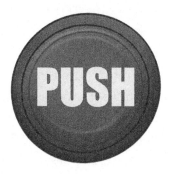

Are you still here?
Great! Now it's time to tackle this head on.

THE SEVEN MINDSETS OF INFERTILITY

Many of us are familiar with the seven stages of grief, especially if we have experienced the loss of a loved one or some other significant trauma. Identifying the different stages of grief and knowing what to expect during each stage can help you understand the emotional changes that occur following a loss. It can also help those around you understand how to support you.

How does this relate to infertility? Certainly, grief can be part of the infertility experience; however applying this same idea to the stages people may go through while trying to conceive provides an interesting framework. It helps us understand ourselves and others who are going through this challenging experience.

When an individual is trying to grow their family, they may move through several mindsets. When they are in one of these mindsets, they are not able to see from a different perspective. They have to go through the experiences related to each mindset to understand it and move to a different one.

What are the Seven Mindsets of Infertility?

1. Believing you can conceive naturally
2. Believing you can conceive with fertility treatment using your own eggs and sperm
3. Choosing to use donor eggs, sperm or embryos
4. Feeling confident that you can carry a pregnancy to term
5. Choosing to engage a surrogate or gestational carrier
6. Exploring other parenting options, such as adoption or fostering
7. Coming to terms with being childless

To be clear, there is no hierarchy to these mindsets. People may not go through them in any particular order and everyone's pathway will be unique depending on their diagnosis and life experiences.

It can explain why people struggling with infertility may become upset when people say things like "Why don't you just adopt?" or "Just relax, and it will happen!" The reason is because they are not in the corresponding mindset to receive that advice. Suggesting that they just relax and it will happen is only relevant in Mindset 1 and advice about adopting is only relevant to those in Mindset 6. Of course, the best option for well-meaning people is to provide no advice at all. Advice giving without being asked is insensitive and shows a lack of understanding of what would truly help someone in one of these Infertility Mindsets.

THE 7 MINDSETS OF INFERTILITY

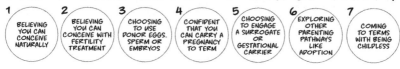

1. BELIEVING YOU CAN CONCEIVE NATURALLY
2. BELIEVING YOU CAN CONCEIVE WITH FERTILITY TREATMENT
3. CHOOSING TO USE DONOR EGGS. SPERM OR EMBRYOS
4. CONFIDENT THAT YOU CAN CARRY A PREGNANCY TO TERM
5. CHOOSING TO ENGAGE A SURROGATE OR GESTATIONAL CARRIER
6. EXPLORING OTHER PARENTING PATHWAYS LIKE ADOPTION
7. COMING TO TERMS WITH BEING CHILDLESS

Understanding the Mindsets of Infertility is useful if:

► You want to understand your partner's behaviour, it can help to know which mindset they are in.
► You are struggling with insensitive things people say, then knowing your current mindset can help you to understand your negative response to unsolicited advice.
► You want to support someone you care about, taking the time to understand which mindset they are in can help you tailor your response to them.

Understanding these mindsets is important within a couple or baby-making team. What happens when you and your partner are not in the same mindset?

Example 1 – Imagine one partner wanting to move on to fertility treatment (Mindset 2) while the other partner is in denial and still believes they can conceive naturally (Mindset 1).

Example 2 – After years of fertility treatment, one partner is ready to move on to Mindset 6 or 7, while the other partner can't move beyond their hope of carrying a pregnancy to term. Acknowledging that you are both seeing your situation from an entirely different perspective can help you be sensitive and understanding to your partner's feelings.

Example 3 – If a couple is undergoing fertility treatment and trying everything they can to conceive with their own eggs and sperm (Mindset 2) it is not an appropriate time for a friend to offer to donate embryos to them. Even though the offer comes from a kind place, it disregards the mindset that the couple is in.

Understanding that other people can be in a different state of mind to you can help you understand their perspective, their comments, or their inability to take action. You can then approach them in a more compassionate way, especially if you don't make them wrong for being in their mindset, just as you are not wrong for being in yours.

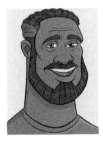

*Our well-meaning friends and family don't know what to say and they put their foot in it more often than not. There's nothing like that unhelpful advice 'have you thought about adopting?' or 'what about an egg donor?' I felt like answering sarcastically. 'Wow, we never thought about that! Thank you so much for that brilliant suggestion.' But I do understand, unless you have been through it, it's hard to understand. - **Michael***

How Will You Know Which Mindset Someone is in?

Ask questions and listen closely to understand their mindset.

- ► What do you think is the best course of action for you right now?
- ► What do you think is the next step for you?
- ► What would like to try now?

You can reflect on these questions for yourself:

- ► What is your mindset at present?
- ► What is your partner's mindset?
- ► What is the mindset of your friends and family?
- ► If someone says something insensitive regarding fertility, what is his or her mindset?
- ► How can you respond with more empathy and kindness, especially if someone you love is not in the same mindset as you?
- ► Which mindset do you need to be in, based on your diagnosis and situation, in order to move forward with living a happy and healthy life? What steps do you need to take to get there?

At some stage, it might be necessary for you to look at your situation and lovingly make a decision that serves both you and your partner. That decision might be to stop treatment and move to the next stage. Part of taking care of your relationship is considering your partner's needs, emotions and desires and deciding together when it is time to move to the next mindset.

If you are anywhere between mindsets 2 and 7, then this book is for you. Read on.

FERTILITY WARRIORS ARE SUPERHEROES

Infertility is incredibly challenging. The medical treatments are gruelling. The waiting is excruciating. The outcomes are often heartbreaking. You may mistakenly assume that while you are going through this difficult process of trying to conceive that you are somehow weak, but you are not, you are a superhero.

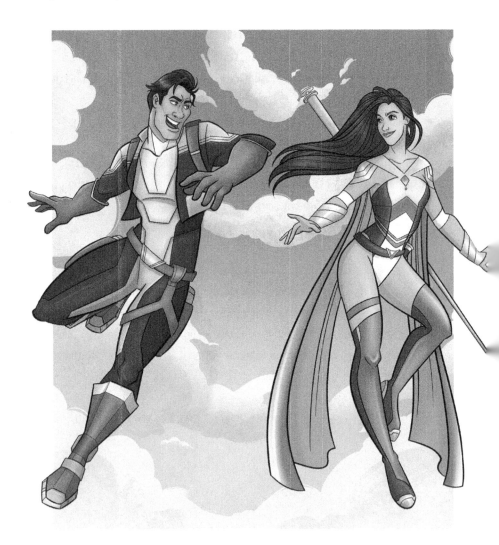

Fertility Warriors and Superheroes Have Secret Identities

A superhero (of any gender) is a character that possesses abilities beyond those of ordinary people. They typically use their powers to help the world become a better place or to achieve an important mission. What greater mission is there than the desire to be a parent and to bring life into the world?

Often the true identity of a superhero is secret. They walk among us in plain clothes and look like regular people in offices and on the streets. Under their clothing, there may be a superhero costume or a collection of bruises from their fertility treatment. Usually, very few people know the identities of superheroes. This is to safeguard them from unwanted attention and to protect their hearts from the wider community, who rarely understand what they're going through.

However, if you look closely, you'll see the secret signs of these superheroes. It might be a white bandage on their elbow from a recent blood test. Maybe they disappear at the strangest moments; you may see a distant look on their face after a pregnancy announcement, or perhaps the smudge of a tear on their cheek from their most recent battle.

They Are Courageous

Just like superheroes, Fertility Warriors face their fears on a daily basis. A superhero is a person who does heroic deeds in a way that a normal person couldn't. Whilst facing infertility, a person develops a particular resilience and the ability to do things they never thought possible, because they are striving towards the thing they so desperately want. Their courage becomes greater than their fear. This is how they build their special powers and abilities. In order to have a true superhero story, there must be a super villain and a super challenge – infertility is certainly that.

They Are Tolerant Of Pain

Superheroes often experience physical discomfort while they are saving the world. Fertility Warriors have a high pain threshold too, that they have developed through a lot of practice. Many endure daily physical pain through injections, swollen ovaries, numerous surgeries and medical procedures. They learn to be tough and to face the pain head on. They know that their mission is more important to them than the avoidance of pain, so they bravely step up every day and get the job done. A good ice pack, heat pack and lots of Band-Aids are necessary tools.

They Do Strange Things With Underpants

Superman wears his underwear on the outside. That's a little strange, but it is just part of being a superhero. Fertility Warriors do strange things with underwear too. They often wear nothing on their bottom half in doctor's offices and fertility clinics and they can make their underwear disappear in a split second, just before the sonographer enters the room.

They May Have A Sidekick Or May Act Alone

Some superheroes have sidekicks, like Batman has Robin. Whether it's a wife, a husband, a partner or a friend, a Fertility Warrior may have a companion in their superhero adventures. Together, they form a unit that is powerful. Each member of the team has times when they are the one saving the day and times when they are the one who needs saving. Their mission is difficult, so they do their best to support each other through it all. A sidekick can double as the designated driver of the Batmobile and maybe even administer an injection or two.

Very special superheroes act alone. They are the bravest and strongest of them all. These lone warriors shoulder tremendous responsibilities and have extra amounts of courage. They are at their best when they are able to complete their mission on their own, and they choose this course of action wholeheartedly.

They May Use Advanced Technology And Medicine To Achieve Their Superhero Status

Some superheroes (for example Batman and Iron Man) derive their status from advanced technology, while others (such as Superman and Spider-Man) possess non-human biology. Fertility Warriors have a team of fertility specialists that help them achieve their superhuman status. While the medications they take are first and foremost to help them conceive, they also help them gain superhuman strength, courage, speed, and agility.

They Are Challenged By Things That Don't Impact Normal People

Just like Superman and kryptonite, they may be momentarily weakened by things that are harmless to other people. A baby shower can leave them breathless; a pregnancy announcement can cause them to cry in their car, an insensitive comment can create great distress. These things may challenge them in a way that doesn't affect regular humans, and it is because they are being called to be so much stronger in so many areas of their lives but they always find a way to keep going.

They Can Complete Superhero Business In Any Private Space

Just like Superman, who changes his clothes in telephone booths, storage rooms, doorways, closets, revolving doors and alleyways, Fertility Warriors can give themselves an injection quickly and efficiently in a public bathroom, car seat or an abandoned office. They can insert a pessary as fast as a speeding bullet. They can run across town and provide a sperm sample in a tiny windowless room. They then return to their desk or whatever else they were doing, as if nothing ever happened, and no one is the wiser.

How They Manage Their Money or Their Job Is Unclear, But They Find A Way

Despite their occasional disappearances to fight crime or go to fertility appointments, superheroes and Fertility Warriors manage to hold down jobs, somehow saving the world and then rushing back to the office to meet their deadlines. Being a superhero isn't cheap (and neither is fertility treatment), but they somehow make it work. Juggling work and finances while going through infertility is very difficult, that is why it takes a superhero to do it.

They Can Be Any Gender, Age, Race Or Sexual Orientation

Superheroes come from a wide array of different backgrounds. Their origin story is part of who they are and it informs how they fight their battles. Fertility Warriors come from many walks of life, and as many of them keep their true identities secret, you can never be sure when you are facing a true fertility hero, regardless of how they look on the outside.

They Have A Sense Of Humour

Whether it's a witty one-liner or clumsy fall, superheroes and Fertility Warriors have the ability to see the lighter side of a tough situation. They have to find ways to laugh or their situation might make them miserable. So, they crack jokes, point out the ridiculousness of what they are experiencing and make their medical team smile.

They Have A Mission and They Are Driven By Love

Every superhero believes in something and wants to fight for it. If Fertility Warriors didn't believe in their dream of growing a family, they would have already given up. They are driven by love. Superheroes can't always win, but they never stop fighting until their story reaches the final destination. They might change their plan or create an alternative ending and they take breaks when they need to recharge their strength; but they keep going until they reach the end of their story.

If you are in the middle of your own trying-to-conceive journey, please hold your head high and give yourself credit, because you are incredible. Next time you walk into a fertility clinic, a baby shower or any place in your Gotham City, walk tall and proud, reminding yourself that YOU ARE AMAZING!

You are a superhero.

YOUR BABY-MAKING TEAM

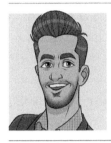

When you have fertility issues, people think that the man should just be strong while the woman experiences all the physical and emotional strain. This is something that people are programmed to believe. We need to reset the thinking around infertility and bring men into the conversation. **- Dr Scott Shemer**

Creating babies is a team sport.

Even if you are planning to raise a child on your own, it still takes a village.

And conception certainly always requires more than one person. At the very least, you need someone to provide sperm, someone to provide an egg, and someone to grow the bun in their oven.

Even if you are lucky enough to be surrounded by supportive friends and family, it really is just the two of you (or three or four of you) who are experiencing infertility. Whether you are using natural conception, intrauterine insemination (IUI), In vitro fertilization (IVF), surrogacy, donor eggs or sperm or adoption, there is a very small group of people who you can call your Baby-Making Team. It might be just you and your partner (wife, girlfriend, husband) or it might include more people, such as your donors, your surrogate, your co-parents or the intended parents.

Whatever your fertility diagnosis, it will soon become obvious that the female partner has the tough end of this deal. Infertility is almost always thought of as a woman's issue, and it's true that women bear the greater burden of it. They are the ones who ultimately either get pregnant or don't, and regardless of which partner has the fertility problem, the woman's body is usually the site of fertility treatment. She will have to undergo more invasive tests, more needles and more procedures. Then, if you're lucky, she will go through the pregnancy and birth. The tests and procedures are pretty invasive, complicated and emotionally draining. Whether you have male or female factor infertility, the 'burden of treatment' will be with her. No matter how badly you want to have a child, her physical and emotional wellbeing is of paramount importance.

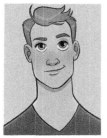

IVF takes a huge physical, hormonal and emotional toll on a woman. Sometimes I felt totally ineffective. I questioned my masculinity, my sense of myself as a man, through those rounds of IVF.

We have to realise that infertility is difficult for men too. During consultations, I felt the conversations were always directed at my wife. I felt like I had to say, 'I'm here too.' I'd deliberately ask a question just to make my presence felt. **- Lucas**

This book is to guide you through your fertility journey. It will explain how to provide the best support to your partner or team. Many people have been through the experience of infertility and have come out the other side. And everybody does get to the other side, in one way or another. The aim is to get through the experience while protecting and nurturing your relationships and the mental health of your entire Baby-Making Team.

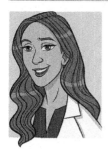

My advice for everyone: ask questions, be patient with the process, take it one hurdle at a time. And BOTH partners need to focus on self-care. Inevitably one partner (typically the one with ovaries and a uterus) is doing more tests, procedures, interventions and it's easy for the other partner to put their own needs last.

We cannot fill from an empty cup; it's important to take care of both partners' needs in the process. **- Dr Lora Shahine**

Let's Talk About It

Let's say that your baby-making team includes yourself and a female partner. Stereotypically, women tend to be very focused on their fertility issues and they want to talk about it all the time. Men tend to push problems they can't immediately solve on to the 'back burner' and they find it difficult to talk about the challenges of conceiving at random times throughout the day.

This can create a frustrating environment where the man feels nagged into talking about infertility all the time and the woman feels unheard, unable to get her needs met and unable to have constructive conversations.

At the end of each chapter, we suggest a Baby-Making Meet Up. It could be like a date night or a meeting. It is a specified amount of time that is set aside when you will talk about your infertility challenges. Make it fun, cook a nice dinner, go to your favourite restaurant, have a walk in the park or visit the beach. The Baby-Making Meet Up should take you outside of your normal daily life and create a clear space for you to focus on the issues, wherever you are in your fertility journey.

Sometimes, your baby-making team will involve more than two people (if you are using donor embryos or a surrogate, for instance). You might be hoping to conceive a child on your own; in that case, we suggest you ask a close friend or family member to support you.

When both partners (or your entire team) know that a Baby-Making Meet Up is scheduled for later in the week, it can put you all at ease. If one partner wants to talk about it often, they can rest assured knowing that they can write their thoughts down and be sure to have the full attention of their partner when discussing them later. If one partner feels overwhelmed by constant fertility talk during the day, they can ask for a break and remind the other partner that they have a Baby-Making Meet Up planned, when they will focus 100 percent of their attention on fertility talk.

It helps all members of your team to be clear about when fertility talk is happening and when it is not.

The Baby-Making Meet Up pages in this book include conversation starters and questions to discuss with your partner or Baby-Making Team. You could write the answers to the questions in a journal to clear your own mind and focus on your fertility goals.

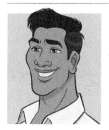

We stuck together through all of those years when we were doing IVF, we were stronger together. **- Thomas**

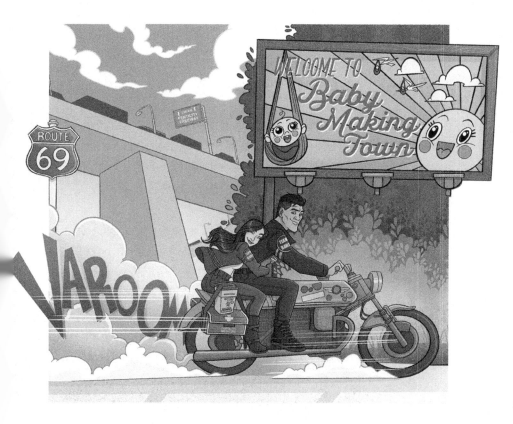

BABY-MAKING MEET UP

Here are some conversation starters for your first baby-making meet up.

▶ Are we committed to this? Let your partner know you are committed to working through your fertility challenges. Ask them if they are also 100 percent committed. Be open to hearing a different perspective.

▶ Do we have the right baby-making team? Do we need to include anyone else?

▶ Which Fertility Mindset are you in? Which Fertility Mindset is your partner in?

THE 7 MINDSETS OF INFERTILITY

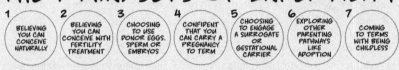

1	2	3	4	5	6	7
BELIEVING YOU CAN CONCEIVE NATURALLY	BELIEVING YOU CAN CONCEIVE WITH FERTILITY TREATMENT	CHOOSING TO USE DONOR EGGS, SPERM OR EMBRYOS	CONFIDENT THAT YOU CAN CARRY A PREGNANCY TO TERM	CHOOSING TO ENGAGE A SURROGATE OR GESTATIONAL CARRIER	EXPLORING OTHER PARENTING PATHWAYS LIKE ADOPTION	COMING TO TERMS WITH BEING CHILDLESS

▶ What do you ultimately want? Take a moment to say out loud to each other why having a family is important to you.

Often people struggling with infertility downplay their dreams, as they are fearful that it will never work out for them. However, to achieve any goal, you have to see an amazing, positive outcome at the end. This is what will give you the motivation to get through the tough challenges ahead.

Even though you know there are challenges ahead, get excited about what a family could look like for you. What kind of parent do you want to be? What activities do you want to do with your children? Why is this important to you?

Remind each other that you are superheroes for embarking on this journey. Although it feels challenging, being brave enough to work through it together proves how strong you are.

See the Baby-Making Meet Up videos and download a workbook at www.InfertilityMan.com/MansGuide

BASIC BIOLOGY

Let's start at the very beginning.

When you were a little kid and you asked: 'Where do babies come from?' you weren't quite given the whole story. 'When a man and a woman love each other very much, they have a special cuddle and then a baby comes out.' Before you had time to say: 'Comes out of what?' the subject was changed.

When you became sexually active, you probably put a lot of effort into *not* getting anyone pregnant. After sniggering through all the serious talks and sex education classes, it seemed like getting a girl pregnant would be really easy. Turns out, it's not always as easy as you thought.

Since you are reading this book, it turns out that it is not at all easy for you.

To understand your specific fertility problem, we need to go back to the beginning and revise the basics of reproduction. It's probably been a while since you had your sex education classes. While I'm sure you have been practicing the act of sex, we need to make sure that we understand the ins and outs of reproduction – which is an entirely different subject altogether.

The first thing you need to know is that men and women are biologically different. Seems obvious, but it is useful to understand how our bodies work in order to create a whole new human.

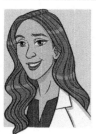

Learning about cycles, ovulation, and overall health is important. We are taught how NOT to conceive very well in health class in school - but we don't learn about hormones, ovaries, and menstrual cycles like we should. **- Dr Lora Shahine**

THE MALE REPRODUCTIVE SYSTEM

Let's start with the male side of the equation.

There is much more to your penis than meets the eye. And your testicles are two incredible units.

The pituitary gland deep within the brainstem tells the testicles to produce sperm-making hormones. One of the hormones produced by the testicles is the famous testosterone. Sperm form inside the testicles and over about two months they mature and move towards the tiny open duct. They sit and wait to be called upon, probably lifting weights and doing push-ups while they bide their time.

When you think about something arousing, or see or feel something arousing, blood flows at a very high pressure down to your penis. Little valves snap shut to trap the blood in there and your penis becomes hard. Believe it or not, there is more to the male reproductive system than the penis, so let's look a little deeper.

When it comes to baby making, your testicles are the most important weapons in your arsenal.

Eight things you need to know about your testicles and sperm

1. The testicles are where your spermatozoa, the male sex cell, is created and stored. This is a major difference between eggs and sperm, while a woman has all her eggs on board before she is even born; men create sperm from scratch throughout their reproductive life.
2. Sperm and semen are different things. Sperm are the little tadpoles that swim to the eggs. Semen is the fluid that contains the sperm. A man can produce a lot of semen with very few sperm or a small amount of semen with loads of sperm.

3. The inner part of the testicles has many small tubes called seminiferous tubules, which are coiled or twisted around. Sperm is made inside these tubules.

4. Your testicles hang away from your body to keep the sperm cool. They need to be lower than body temperature to survive, so the dangling is to prevent things from getting too warm down there. Keeping your testicles separate from your body is a way of keeping them nicely air-conditioned. They pull up inside your body when it's cold because that helps to keep the temperature exactly where it needs to be. The cremasteric muscle contracts to pull them in and relaxes to let them dangle, this is called the cremasteric reflex.

5. Stress can also make the cremasteric reflex work. If a male human or mammal gets into a fight, then its testicles are in danger so they automatically pull up close to the body. The cremasteric reflex happens during sexual intercourse as well.

6. It may help your fertility if you keep your scrotum cool. If you wear tight underwear, sit with a computer on your lap, have hot baths, jump in a hot spa or sauna, then your overheated sperm won't be coming out of there alive. With everything you are going through trying to conceive this baby, it's important to keep them cool.

7. When a man feels sexual desire, sperm cells go through the ejaculatory duct. They are combined with liquid called seminal fluid from a gland called the prostate. The prostate has muscles that push the sperm and fluid into the urethra.

8. During sexual intercourse, seminal fluid containing the sperm comes out through the urethral opening when a man ejaculates.

So now that we have that sorted, let's look at the other side of the baby-making equation.

THE FEMALE REPRODUCTIVE SYSTEM

An epic quest for sperm.

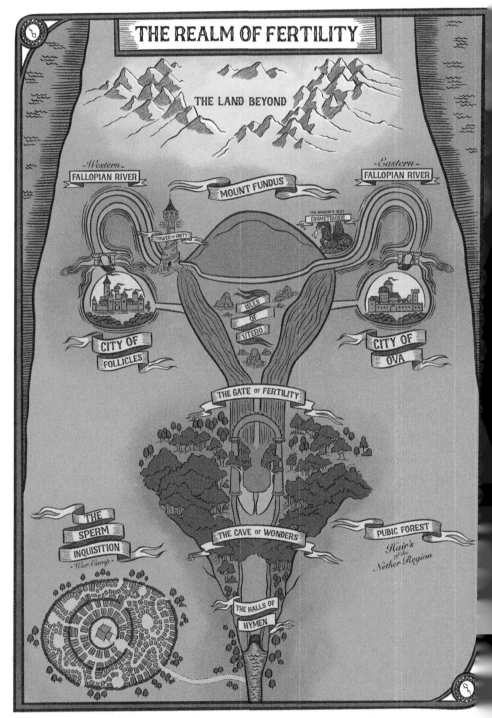

The 10 Hurdles of the Female Reproductive System

Sperm make quite a voyage in order to fertilise an egg. Many of them will not survive the journey, but you can come through unscathed if you take the time to prepare yourself for the battle that lies ahead.

The sperm travel about 15 to 18 centimetres from the vagina to the egg. As sperm are only 1/600 millimetres in length, this is equivalent to a grown man swimming from Melbourne to Perth in total darkness. It is quite a trek for these little guys.

1. The vagina. The first obstacle for sperm is getting inside a vagina.
2. Once they are inside, they are in a hostile environment. The vagina is naturally acidic, one of nature's ways of weeding out the good sperm from the bad. One function of semen is to neutralise some of that acidity, but still almost immediately about 40 million sperm are slaughtered by this natural acidity – it's a massacre.
3. The woman's white blood cells attack sperm. They are killers, highly trained to attack anything foreign to the woman's body and your sperm. Usually it's a good thing when white blood cells attack foreign bacteria, but it's not helpful for your sperm soldiers, so a few more will be killed.
4. The cervix. Next, the sperm find themselves at the cervix, a tight muscular piece of tissue that acts as a gateway between the vagina and the uterus.
5. The uterus. Once they have slipped past the cervix, the sperm enter the uterus. More sperm will fall at this stage, some will run out of energy, stop swimming and die, and others will simply swim the wrong way. On average, only about 1,000 will make it anywhere near the egg.
6. At the top of the uterus, the teeny tiny eggs live in follicles, which are like little water balloons in each of the ovaries. They have lived in the ovaries since before the woman was even born. Unfortunately, from then on, through the menstrual cycle the number of eggs just keeps reducing and reducing until there are no eggs left suitable for reproduction.

7. Timing. Once a month, one of the ovaries releases an egg, sending it down the connecting fallopian tube toward the uterus, so the sperm must arrive at a good time, during the woman's 'fertile window'.

8. The fallopian tube. The sperm sneak up the fallopian tube to meet the egg coming from the other direction.

9. The egg. The remaining sperm that have made it this far attack the egg and try to squeeze inside. Only one will make it. Victory! Once that valiant sperm is inside, the egg will activate her defences and shut out the rest of the sperm.

10. Fertilisation. With the sperm inside, the egg transforms into an embryo. This means that the single cell starts to divide and multiply itself to form more and more cells.

11. Implantation. The embryo continues the journey down the fallopian tube and lands in the uterus where it attaches itself to the wall, otherwise known as the endometrium.

So many things can go wrong during this long journey to fertilisation. Too few sperm, low-quality sperm, issues with ovulation, low-quality eggs, scarring or cysts in the fallopian tubes that prevent the egg from meeting the sperm or the embryo failing to implant inside the uterus. Genetic problems can also cause infertility. Even just getting the timing wrong will prevent a baby from being created. That's why we need to understand the menstrual cycle.

The Period

Period talk may have been something you avoided in the past. However, now that you are a grown man trying to have a baby, there is no avoiding it any longer. Having some understanding of the menstrual cycle is only going to help this process, both for conceiving and for supporting your partner.

The first thing to realise is that the period is only one part of a woman's cycle, which is actually made up of different phases. At each phase, hormones are released, which cause the changes to take place. An average menstrual cycle lasts between 25 days and 31 days, it can vary and some women have very irregular cycles.

The Menstrual Cycle

A cycle takes place in two main areas; in the ovaries with the production of eggs and in the uterus as it prepares for a potential pregnancy.

CYCLE	PRE-OVULATION		OVULATION	POST-OVULATION
OVARIAN CYCLE	FOLLICULAR PHASE			LUTEAL PHASE
UTERINE CYCLE	MENSTRUAL	PROLIFERATIVE		SECRETORY

1. The Follicular phase

The follicular phase is the first part of the ovarian cycle. Tiny follicles inside the ovaries mature and get ready to release an egg. Several follicles will enlarge, but only one of them will win the battle to be the dominant follicle. It usually takes about 10 to 14 days to mature the egg.

Menstruation

Meanwhile, in the uterus, menstruation (also called menstrual bleeding, menses or a period) is taking place. Day 1 of the period is the first day of a whole new menstrual cycle. The period normally serves as a sign that a woman has not become pregnant during the previous month.

Proliferative phase

The proliferative phase is the second phase of the uterine cycle when oestrogen causes the lining of the uterus to grow, or proliferate, to get ready in case there is a pregnancy during this month.

2. Ovulation

In this phase, a mature egg is released from the ovarian follicles and is sent down the fallopian tubes. On rare occasions, two or three are released, potentially causing twins or triplets. If there are any sperm in the woman's uterus at this time, this is when the egg and sperm will meet.

3. The Luteal phase

The luteal phase is the final part of the cycle, when the hormones do all kinds of crazy stuff to finish everything off. Over about two weeks, the empty follicle transforms into a structure known as the corpus luteum. This structure releases progesterone, along with small amounts of oestrogen.

Secretory phase

In the uterus, the endometrium (the lining of the uterus) has become recep-tive to the implantation of the blastocyst (otherwise known as the embryo, the egg and the sperm together) and supportive of an early pregnancy. This has the side effect of raising the woman's basal body temperature.
Finally, falling levels of progesterone trigger menstruation and the beginning of the next cycle.

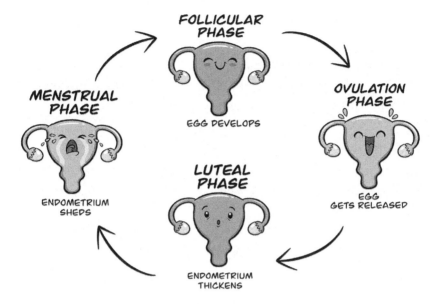

FOLLICULAR
PHASE

EGG DEVELOPS

OVULATION
PHASE

EGG
GETS RELEASED

MENSTRUAL
PHASE

ENDOMETRIUM
SHEDS

LUTEAL
PHASE

ENDOMETRIUM
THICKENS

So what does all this mean for you?

Simply put, Day 1 of her cycle is the first day of 'full flow' of her period. The words 'full flow' are important, in most cases, you begin a fertility treatment when the period is in full swing, not just 'spotting'. Her period lasts for between 1 and 5 days, every woman is different. The period is her uterus doing a bit of a spring clean, clearing out the old endometrial lining to prepare a fresh uterus lining in case a pregnancy starts next month.

It might be nice to ask your partner how long her cycle usually lasts. If you are going to be doing fertility treatment, or if you are just trying to have sex at the optimal time for conception, you are going to need to know. It is best to get ahead and ask your partner to share this kind of info with you. She is going to feel more supported than if she feels like she has to hassle you about it.

Better yet, there are some really great apps where a woman can track her cycle and even share it to an app on your phone – that can really cut down the need for lots of period conversations.

Fertilisation and Implantation

Here is what is supposed to happen next …
The egg and the sperm have hooked up with each other and, in that instant, they create the hereditary characteristics of a new individual.

It goes like this:
Fertilisation – The egg and sperm fuse into a new cell called a zygote with distinctive genetic information. The unique DNA blueprint of a human has been established.

After Twelve Hours – The first cell divides into two. Each cell divides again about every 24 hours through a process called mitosis.

After Two Days – The embryo now has four to eight cells. It's still in the fallopian tube, but it's making its way to the uterus. The cells continue to divide and multiply.

After Five Days – The cluster of about 100 cells is now called a blastocyst. Its aim now is to move down the fallopian tube and then to attach itself to the wall of the uterus.

Note: if the embryo gets stuck in the fallopian tube, this becomes an ectopic pregnancy, which can be dangerous to the woman and she will need medical care.

After Eight to Ten Days – The blastocyst has attached to a spot on the wall of the uterus. The embryo secretes hCG, and the uterus receives the signal not to menstruate this month.

After Twelve Days – The amniotic sac is formed, which is where the baby will live for the next nine months.

After Two Weeks – If an embryo has implanted and is growing, a pregnancy has begun. Your doctor will probably schedule a blood test 10 to 14 days after the embryo transfer. The blood test will detect and measure the hormone hCG, the 'pregnancy hormone.'

If a pregnancy has not begun, a menstrual period will soon begin, starting a whole new menstrual cycle.

DAY 0	EGG RETRIEVAL AND INSEMINATION	
DAY 1	FERTILISATION	
DAY 2	CLEAVAGE STAGE (4 CELLS)	
DAY 3	CLEAVAGE STAGE (8 CELLS)	
DAY 4	MORULA STAGE	
DAY 5+	BLASTOCYST STAGE	
	BLASTOCYST STAGE/ HATCHING STAGE	

TRYING TO CONCEIVE NATURALLY

So, you and your partner are trying to get pregnant. If you're hoping to conceive naturally, you're having sex regularly, but every month, her period starts.

In the beginning, when you think you'll get pregnant right away, it's good sex. And it's great not having to worry about protection. Each time you have sex, you wonder if you have conceived.

Then several months go by and you realise that she's not getting pregnant.

Over time, believe it or not, having sex at specified times could feel a bit like a chore. Your partner's usual coy question "Shall we go to bed?" turns into "Alright, fine, let's get this over with!" If you have to do baby-making sex, be proud of yourself, because it's not always easy.

This is where you really get a chance to shine. Bring some fun and spontaneity to the process. Make her laugh, compliment her, tease her, flirt with her just like you did when you first got together. Flirt like your life depended on it! Sex begins outside the bedroom (especially for the ladies) so pay conscious attention to keeping the spark alive in your relationship, since you have to have sex anyway, do your very best to make it fun and loving.

As time passes and no pregnancy occurs, you both may start to feel the pressure.

She might start doing things like:

- ► Making requests for sex when she is ovulating (that might not seem very sexy)
- ► Changing her diet
- ► Suggesting you change your diet
- ► Noticing phantom symptoms, hoping she might be pregnant
- ► Crying when she gets her period

With each month that passes, this can become more and more upsetting. If you are trying to get pregnant naturally, your partner needs your support now more than ever. As a team, you can both pay closer attention to her cycle, to make sure that you are trying to conceive on her most fertile days of each month.

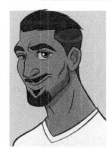

*When we got married, we decided we would just wait a few years. We weren't in a rush, we were focused on our careers. We would talk about what our dream of the future was, little things like what kind of car we would need to fit our kids and where we would take our kids on family holidays, things like that. We never talked about what would happen if one of us couldn't have kids. Then we came off birth control and we thought maybe something would happen... and nothing ever did. - **Justin***

CHARTING

The exact time that your partner ovulates depends on the length of her cycle. The typical day of ovulation for many women is Day 14 (that is two weeks after Day 1 of her period). So, lots of couples have sex on Days 12, 13 and 14 because sperm can stay alive in the system for up to four days. But what happens if she doesn't ovulate on Day 14? What if she has an irregular cycle or just naturally ovulates earlier or later each month?

This is where charting becomes really useful. If she can work out over a few months when she usually ovulates by keeping track of it, then that will help make sure you do the baby-making deed on the right days. Your female counterpart will need to record the data relating to her menstrual cycle, but it is important that you know a little about how it works. Your job is to give her as much support as she needs.

There are a few things going on in her body that she will keep track of:
1. Her period. This one is pretty obvious; she will keep track of which days she has her period and how heavy or light the flow is.
2. Her temperature. She will keep track of her 'basal body temperature', which means she will take her temperature first thing every morning. After she ovulates, the hormones that go rushing through her body, in particular progesterone, raise her body temperature between 0.4 and 0.8 degrees. Once her temperature goes up, it's already too late. The reason to keep track of it is so that she has a good chance of estimating when she will ovulate *next month*.
3. Cervical mucus. She is going to keep track of what is going on in her underwear. In the days leading up to ovulation, your partner's cervix will produce mucus, which will help the sperm make their journey. It becomes thicker and stickier and can be compared to raw egg white.
4. Ovulation prediction. Using tests she can purchase, she may pee on some sticks that will tell her when she is close to ovulating. The tests measure surges in luteinising hormone, which is the one that triggers ovulation.

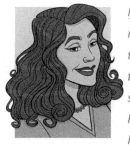

If her temperature goes up, you have already missed the window. You need to have sex before her temperature goes up. A lot of the period apps and trackers are inaccurate. Charting is great for getting a sense of her cycle and making sure it is pretty regular, however, seeking medical advice sooner rather than later is always a good option.

*If her cycle is shorter than 24 days or longer than 35 days, chances are there is a problem and she definitely needs to get her egg bank evaluated and make sure she is ovulating. - **Dr Lynn Burmeister***

Your partner is most likely well versed in all of this, but if she isn't, at least you know a little to point her in the right direction. There are loads of websites and apps that she can use to chart her cycle and many of them can share this info directly to your phone.

As always, even though charting is mostly her thing, show your support. You will have to get involved when it is time to 'do the deed', so paying attention to the schedule is very helpful.

It is better to have a rough idea of when you're going to be having sex from an app, rather than a stressed-out woman demanding that you have sex 'right now' as then the two of you can pretend to be a bit more spontaneous.

Over time, some couples find baby-making sex a little stressful. You should have a frank discussion about what would work best for the two of you as a couple. Perhaps you would rather not know when she is ovulating, in order to help sex feel more spontaneous? Or you might like to have the information in your calendar. You can do this using an online calendar or an app. A paper calendar hung on the wall works perfectly well too. Or you may prefer not to know when the best time for 'baby dancing' will be and for her to just let you know when she is in the mood.

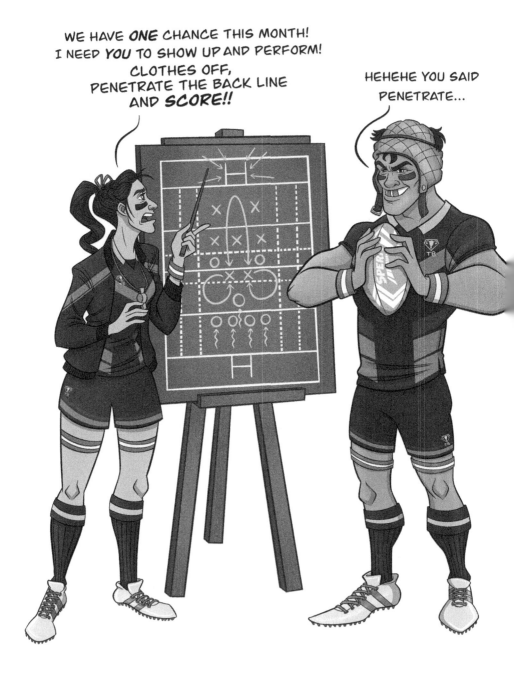

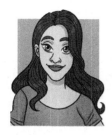

FROM LAURA

For the ladies

I just wanted to take a quick moment to say hello to any women reading this book.

Welcome! Hopefully there will be lots of info here that is useful to you too. I know you are probably reading this to gain some insight into your partner's experience of infertility. Everyone processes things differently, so it is difficult to truly understand what it feels like for another person. However, I believe your partner feels things just as deeply as you do, though he may express it differently.

My biggest piece of advice: tell him what you need and what you want. A good man genuinely wants to support you, but no one can read your mind. Be clear about how he can take care of you during this challenging time. Infertility is difficult enough already, so make it easy for him to help you.

Take care of him too. We have met so many men through our Infertility Man online channels who feel the emotions of infertility so deeply and they would give anything to have the family of your dreams with you.

BABY-MAKING MEET UP

It's time to embark on an information-gathering mission. The first step is for you and your Baby-Making Team (you and your partner, or anyone else involved) to get on the same page.

It's time to ask some questions. Even if you think you know the answers, ask these questions anyway. You might surprise yourself and learn something new.

Both
▶ Do you have any diagnosed conditions that may affect your fertility?
▶ Do you have any concerns about your fertility?

Him
▶ Have you had a semen test before?

Her
▶ Talk about her menstrual cycle.
▶ How many days does it usually go for?
▶ When will be Day 1 of her next cycle?
▶ When is she expecting to get her period? Mark this on your schedule.
▶ Is her cycle regular and the same each month?
▶ How does she track her period? Does she use a diary or an app?
▶ How will you share information about her cycle?

Talk about baby-making sex.
▶ How do you both feel about planning sex around fertile days?
▶ How do you prefer for your partner to initiate sex?
▶ Is there anything that each of you could do to make it easier or more enjoyable?

Discuss how long you will continue trying to conceive naturally.
▶ Is there anything you need to change?
▶ Is there anything different you could try?
▶ When will you seek medical advice?

See the Baby-Making Meet Up videos and download a workbook at www.InfertilityMan.com/MansGuide

FROM JON

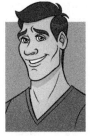

Years ago, I had health challenges that lead to my infertility.

Eight years before we needed IVF, I was on holiday in Fiji, blissfully unaware that my life was about to change. I was feeling a weird pain sensation in my groin area. Guys, you all know what it is like to be kicked in the balls. This was how it felt, and it was constant. A relentless, gnawing feeling that I could not shake, no matter what I did. Stretching, showering and swimming did not relieve this pain. My right testicle felt different, hard, and a little bigger than its friend next door. I ignored it, thinking 'Ah well, it'll be alright.'

I finally decided I would see my doctor on my return to Australia, and in good old bloke style, I put off my appointment until the pain became absolutely unbearable. I arrived early to my appointment and sat uncomfortably in the waiting area. The doctor ushered me into his examination room. I told him about the pain, the tenderness and the odd shape of my right testicle. After examining me, the doctor said, 'I am certain it is epididymitis, but to be sure you should go to see a specialist and have an ultrasound.' I thought it best to get it done sooner rather than later (the first intelligent thought so far).

I quickly set up an appointment with an urologist. The first thing he did was an ultrasound. He checked the good testicle for comparison and then went a little quiet, having moved over to my sore one. He said plainly, 'Do you want me to show you now?' 'Yeah, go for it mate' I said and he turned the monitor to face me. All I saw was a mish mash of blue and red blotches. He showed me the good testicle and then moved to the other one, which had basically become a tumour.

I left with my head in a spin. I went home and contemplated what might happen next. Scary stuff, if you think about it, such a change of pace from the carefree holiday I had just returned from.

The next six days were a blur, a doctor's appointment, a specialist urologist appointment the following day, CT scans and bloods the day after that, then a call from the specialist's office booking me in for surgery on the coming Monday.

HOLY BALLS. This got real very quickly!

An interesting aside, my urologist never mentioned the word cancer. When explaining it, he said it was a non-seminoma and it needed to come out. He said, 'I think you should see my mate', who later we found out to be an oncologist, but still no mention of the C-word.

I went in for the surgery and had my right testicle removed. They offered me the option to have a prosthetic ball put in place. I accepted without much knowledge of what it would feel like afterwards. Post-surgery, it's strange to live with this foreign object between my legs. It has become quite the encumbrance and never goes where I want it to go.

I had continuous monitoring of my blood, chest, abdomen and pelvis for the next five years. I was given the 'all clear' and have not looked back since.

Though it may sound cliché, this experience really changed my life. It set in motion some massive life changes and a move toward an even better health and exercise regime. It was not all plain sailing, but this experience made me committed to taking care of my health. I spent the next few years trying out different lifestyle changes (Blood Type, Keto, High Protein, Low Carb and supplements) with the best results coming from a whole food plant-based diet. There are loads of animals happy that I no longer eat them. The big C created a change in me and a new energy towards life.

Years later. I was driving and listening to a book called The Gratitude Effect, by Dr John DeMartini. Having always wondered why cancer came into my life, a particular quote from the book stood out to me.

"Life is happening for us, not to us."

Life gave me cancer because there were areas of my life that I was not paying attention to. Cancer caused me to change my direction; at a fundamental level, it was change or die.

Going to see a doctor when things don't feel right is something that men tend to postpone. I am so glad that I did eventually go to see a doctor and thank goodness I didn't leave it any longer.

Certainly when the time came to have my fertility checked out, I didn't waste a moment. I hope my story encourages you to take immediate action for yourself.

SEEING THE DOCTOR

After months of trying, one of you has suggested that making a baby may require the assistance of a professional. This is the first step of moving into Mindset 2, coming to understand that you might need medical assistance to conceive.

The standard recommendation is that you should have fertility testing after one year of having unprotected sex or six months if she is over 35 years old. That is the recommendation, but here is another perspective – why not find out what is happening sooner rather than later?

Making progress is always going to feel better than getting stuck with no information. You will feel more in control of your situation if you take action.

Dr Lynn Burmeister is a renowned fertility specialist in Melbourne, Australia. She has over 20 years experience in obstetrics and fertility and is the owner and medical Director at No. 1 Fertility. She explains why pre-pregnancy checks are so important.

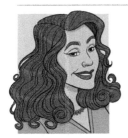

They say, if you are under 35, then you should start fertility testing when you have been trying to conceive for a year, but that doesn't really make sense. You could try for a year and then find out you have no sperm or she's not ovulating! So maybe we should normalise going to your doctor for a pre-pregnancy consultation. It doesn't need to be a fertility specialist, it could be an obstetrician or even a GP. There are things you should check out before you try to have a baby, for example:

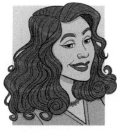

- Ovulation and egg reserve

- Sperm analysis.

- Basic pelvic assessments and ultrasounds to check that there is nothing inside the uterus, ovaries or testicles that might stop you from getting pregnant.

*- Genetic Screening, to make sure that neither of you are carrying a gene that could make your baby unwell. I believe it is important to have these checks before you waste an entire year, even if you're young. Before you start trying to conceive, you should start taking prenatal vitamins as well. When you are thinking about getting pregnant, you need a good pre-pregnancy consultation. - **Dr Lynn Burmeister***

We have never spoken to an infertile couple who wishes they had waited longer to seek medical attention. The longer you leave it, the more it becomes a race against the clock later in the process.

As men, we generally like to be able to fix things ourselves. We don't like to stop and ask for directions. We may not want to face up to reality, especially if we're a little worried that reality might be something we are not ready to deal with. If you are taking the time to read these words, then you are ready to face this challenge. Your way of facing this situation and providing for your future family is to get checked out now.

Imagine it like a little light suddenly popping up on the dashboard of your car. At first it might have been orange, but right now it is flashing red. You wouldn't want to further damage your car by leaving it any longer, right? You know that the earlier you take the car to the mechanic to have a look under the hood, the more likely that you are going to diagnose the problem and get it fixed before it causes further damage. If you are reading this book, then the red light on your fertility is flashing, and it is time to seek some answers.

Don't leave this up to your partner. Don't make her have to nag you. Be first to suggest to her that it is time to get tested. Book the doctor's appointment for yourself. Take action now. Put this book down and pick up your phone or your computer and book a doctor's appointment right now.

If you can't book online, set an alarm to remind you to book during business hours. Talk to your partner. Help her book an appointment to see a doctor too.

Have you done it?

Don't read any further until you have.

Burying your head in the sand will not make this problem go away, so get out in front of it and get the process started.

OK, now that you've taken that step, don't you feel better? Taking action always feels better than just thinking about it.

Just seeking some medical advice may remove some of the worry for you and your partner. It will help her relax and feel more certain that you have started to get some help, so she won't need to worry in silence. Why wait for 6 or 12 months when you can take some of that pressure off now?

STEP 1
SEEING YOUR GENERAL PRACTITIONER

When you have your first appointment with your general practitioner (or primary care physician or family doctor), be prepared for some personal questions. The doctor may ask about any sexually transmitted diseases either of you may have or had in the past. They may ask about any previous pregnancies that either of you has been involved in and what happened with those pregnancies, including if they were aborted. If there is anything you think you should share with your partner (or that they should share with you), it might be a good idea to do this in private before the appointment rather than wait to disclose it in front of your doctor.

Your doctor may ask you about your sex life, so be prepared to share some information that you don't normally share. Remember, your doctor is unlikely to be shocked; they have heard it all before and have had this conversation many times. This is the first of many confidential conversations you will have if you are going to continue with fertility treatment and hopefully have a baby one day.

If you visit a GP and they tell you to just go away and keep trying, insist that they investigate further or go to see another doctor. We want to normalise the urge to see a fertility specialist sooner rather than later. Many couples are turned away by doctors saying, 'time is on your side, try to relax, give it time.' If you are concerned enough to visit a doctor, then you should have your concerns heard. If a GP is unwilling to listen to you and help you get tested, then they are not the doctor you need. Find another doctor who is willing to work with you. Seeking second opinions and essentially 'firing' doctors who didn't listen to your concerns is a good strategy as you find out more about your infertility diagnosis.

Your GP can arrange a few tests that are not expensive or invasive. You could do them as soon as possible. All it takes is a bit of mental gymnastics to be honest with yourself and admit that it is time to seek a medical opinion.

Dr Darren Katz is a urologist and male fertility microsurgeon who serves as Medical Director of Men's Health Melbourne. He explains why it is so important for men to be tested at the same time as their female counterpart.

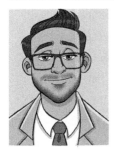

When a couple comes in for infertility, you'll see that the woman has gone through the ringer, she has had all the tests to try to figure out why the couple is not conceiving. Then suddenly they think 'well maybe we'll check him?' Lo and behold, there is the problem.
*My suggestion is if your partner is getting a test, then you need a test too. It's as simple as a blood test and a semen analysis. If those are ok, then you're pretty good to go, but if not, then you will need further testing. It's really, really important. Both the male and female partners need to be assessed at the same time; the male needs to be looked at as well. It shouldn't be an afterthought. - **Dr Darren Katz**

Your GP may set up some simple blood and urine tests, or perhaps even a sperm test for you and pelvic ultrasound for her. Your partner may have her anti-Müllerian hormone (AMH) levels checked, which will give you a very basic insight into her egg reserves. Don't freak out if your preliminary sperm and AMH tests reveal an issue you weren't expecting. It is still early days and there is more to learn about your diagnosis.

While you're with the doctor, you could ask them to set up the standard testing that is good to do before any pregnancy such as STDs, HIV, Syphilis, Chlamydia, Hepatitis, Rubella (German measles) and Varicella (chicken pox). Also ask to get some general health tests done at the same time, such as iron and vitamin levels, thyroid function and anything else your doctor can check for you. You will end up doing this for your fertility specialist anyway, so best to get a head start. Or your GP may refer you directly to a fertility clinic.

STEP 2
CHOOSING YOUR FERTILITY SPECIALIST

It's unlikely that you will know much about the fertility doctors in your area at the beginning. Usually, patients end up seeing a particular specialist because they are referred to them by their GP.

FROM JON

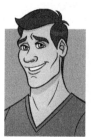

I picked our first fertility doctor by looking at a map and choosing the clinic closest to our house. It was literally walking distance from where we lived. I had looked at the photos of the doctors on their website and I chose the one that I thought looked good - I don't know what I based that decision on. When I called the clinic, that doctor wasn't available so, they randomly assigned me to another one. Clearly, this was not a very careful selection process. As we were at the beginning of our fertility journey, we didn't know any better. We met with the doctor and started the initial testing.

The first procedure I had was called a Fine Needle Aspiration. The doctor inserts a needle into the testicle and then draws back the plunger of the syringe, hoping to extract some sperm. The first pass came up with nothing, the second pass came up with nothing, and then the doctor asked if we wanted to try one more time. Laura and I looked at each other and thought there was nothing to lose, so we did one more pass.

The doctor looked at me in that moment and said, "Geez, you're a braver man than me, I couldn't do this." That comment was surprising to me, as he stuck me with the needle one more time. It was on this third pass of the needle that we found one sperm and it was immotile, meaning it was not swimming at all. The doctor told us we might find more in a sperm retrieval surgery. We were over the moon, even though there was just one sperm. We were excited because we believed that where there was one, there could be more.

The next step was our first IVF cycle. Laura began injecting follicle-stimulating hormones and on Day 9 of her cycle she went to have an ultrasound to see how her ovaries were responding. She called me from the doctor's office in tears. She was upset because the scan showed only six follicles, so only six potential eggs. We now know that this is a reasonably good number (and we know that other people often get fewer or none at all). However, Laura was expecting more, at least 20, so she was disappointed and upset. In hindsight, I should have gone to the appointment with her. From then on, I always made myself available for the first follicle scan of each cycle.

The doctor suggested that we cancel this cycle because of the low number of follicles. We were intending for me to have my sperm retrieval surgery (microTESE) on the same day as Laura's egg retrieval. With only six follicles (and probably fewer eggs), it didn't seem that we would be successful. We were shocked that it hadn't worked out. We cancelled the cycle. At the time, we considered this a 'bad day' in our fertility journey.

It is interesting how sometimes your worst days can turn out to be your best. It was soon evident that our first doctor wasn't experienced in handling a very specialised case like ours. On his advice, we would have gone into my microTESE with very few fresh eggs. Embryos are much more stable for freezing and thawing than sperm on their own (especially my poor-quality sperm). The safest way for my sperm to be frozen would be inside Laura's eggs as embryos. If we had gone ahead with only using a few fresh eggs, our fertility treatment would most likely have been unsuccessful. And you can really only do the microTESE procedure once. What we needed was a large number of frozen eggs as well as some fresh eggs before my sperm retrieval. We would have blown our chance of conceiving my biological child forever.

When Laura had so few follicles, we thought it was a bad day. Looking back, thank goodness it didn't go as we wanted.

We didn't know any of this at the time, so we went back to the clinic in search of answers. It really felt as though we weren't important to them; we were just a number, another patient. The doctor really didn't have any solutions for us and dismissed our questions without providing answers. At the time, I remember I was furious and I know that Laura says that it's the only time she has seen me mad. She thought I was going to punch the doctor. I wasn't going to, but I was certainly annoyed.

In the end, it was a blessing that this first cycle didn't work out. The experience highlighted that no one was going to care about our fertility treatment more than us, not even our doctor. That is also true for you. This is not to say that medical staff aren't caring people, it is just a fact that you care more about your fertility treatment than anyone else. No one will ever care as much as you, so you are the person who needs to drive your treatment, to be informed and to make the important decisions.

Not all doctors are equally skilled, as with any profession, some are better than others. They each have different experience levels, areas of expertise, and bedside manners. Fertility clinics vary greatly in their prices and facilities, so you might find a better deal by shopping around. Selecting a fertility specialist may be one of the most important decisions in your quest to have a baby. While it may work out ok to let your GP choose for you, you might also decide to do some research in order to find the best specialist for your situation. Do your research, read the reviews, ask questions and make a careful, considered decision.

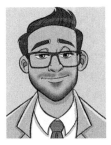 *As with most procedures and surgery, there is experience and a learning curve. I published a paper with my team looking at my own learning curve for microTESE in the last five years and I have improved my outcomes. My success rate was about 40% earlier on in my experience and it has increased to over 60% success rate for finding sperm. So even in my personal experience, I know that you just get better. And it is not just me, this is a team effort, there are the IVF specialists and the team in the IVF lab. Those hard working embryologists who spend hours and hours back in the lab searching through all the tissue that I have given them, trying to find that one little wriggler that they can inject into the egg. So the success rate also comes from the IVF lab's learning curve too. Make sure that you are linked to a great clinic and that they have the experience and the expertise of the lab behind them as well. It is truly a joint team effort when there is success.*

- Dr Darren Katz

THINGS TO LOOK FOR IN A FERTILITY CLINIC

There are many things to consider when choosing a fertility clinic and a good one should give you the opportunity to ask questions before you begin.

Find out more:
- ► Go to information nights
- ► Check out their website
- ► Follow your doctor or clinic on social media
- ► Ask for an information pack
- ► Have an initial consultation with the doctor (although be aware this may attract a cost)
- ► Visit the clinics in person

Remember, you will most likely be paying them a lot of money in the future, so make sure you feel good about your decision. Don't rush into it without doing some research.

Check online discussions and social media groups in your area. Keep in mind that reviews may be skewed by the outcome of the writer (whether or not they were successful in having a baby). Better still, ask people you know who have had fertility treatment. It's amazing how many people you know (or friends of friends) who have done IVF, once you ask around.

Find out about the clinic's policies, procedures and the way they care for their patients from people who have already used them. Ensuring that their bedside manner is compatible with your needs is essential for a good experience.

FROM LAURA

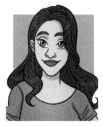

I think there might be an innate quality in many dads (and dads-to-be) that drives them to want to provide and protect. Having the right car seat correctly fitted and a good sturdy pram is important to them to keep their baby safe.

Even though your babies aren't born yet, your choice of fertility doctor is something you should think about carefully. This is the first chance you have to provide for your children and begin protecting them before they are even born. The right doctor can ensure the safety of your future family and your partner. Fertility treatment can be a very expensive purchase and should be treated as such, particularly when it comes to doing the research. As a woman, I would feel so protected and cared for if my man was actively engaged in choosing the fertility clinic, if he made a spreadsheet, compared prices and looked at success rates. Then, like with other big purchases in our life, it would be lovely if he narrowed it down to a shortlist and made the final decision with me. It would make me feel as though we were part of a team.

Tip: Many fertility doctors have long waiting lists, especially the really great ones. Make some calls early and get on the waiting lists at a few clinics and then, if you decide on a particular doctor, you can always cancel unnecessary appointments.

FERTILITY CLINIC CHECKLIST

You will most likely spend quite a bit of time at your fertility clinic, so here are some things to consider.

Important: *The list below is very comprehensive and could be overwhelming. You should look through and decide which points are most important to you and focus on those. You don't need to tick off every item on the list.*

Doctor

▶ Does the doctor have an excellent reputation?

▶ Do they have good online reviews?

▶ Do people speak well of them in IVF social media groups?

▶ Do they have expertise in your particular fertility issue?

▶ Will the doctor perform all the procedures? If not, who will?

▶ Do you feel comfortable with them?

Nurses and Staff

If you are doing IVF or other fertility treatments, you will deal with the nurses potentially more often than your doctor.

▶ Do you like the energy of the clinic?

▶ Will you be able to speak directly with the embryologist? (See glossary)

▶ Do the staff have good reviews?

▶ Do they have a positive and friendly attitude?

▶ Do you feel comfortable with the nurses?

Success Rates

▶ Ask for some information on the clinic's success rate.

▶ Ask about their pregnancy rate and their live birth rate.

Be sure to determine whether your doctor is talking about pregnancy rates or live birth rates when discussing specific treatments so you can make accurate comparisons. For example, a treatment may have a 30 percent pregnancy rate per cycle but only a 25 percent live birth rate because of miscarriages.

Location

- ▶ How far is the clinic from your home?
- ▶ Is parking available?
- ▶ Do they have several locations?
- ▶ Where do they perform the procedures?
- ▶ Where do they store eggs, sperm and embryos?

Flexibility

- ▶ How available will the staff be during your cycle?
- ▶ Are they available on weekends and public holidays?
- ▶ On which dates are they closed during the year and will this affect your treatment?
- ▶ Some clinics only do IVF egg retrievals and transfers on some days of the week, so ask about this too.

Cost

- ▶ Ask for a list of all the potential costs.
- ▶ Ask about government rebates. Do you qualify for financial support?
- ▶ Does your health insurance cover some costs?
- ▶ Pay close attention for unexpected extras.
- ▶ Do they offer complimentary services such as acupuncture, massage, and nutritional advice, and do these have an additional cost?

Medicines

► How much are you expecting to pay for medicines?
► Are you able to shop around for the drugs or does your clinic only offer one pharmacy option?

Males

► Get a sense of how men are treated in the clinic. Are men ignored or included?
► How do they take care of their male clients?
► What facilities do they have for men, for example, the sperm collection rooms?
► Do they allow you to produce your sperm sample at home and bring it in?
► If you need a procedure to retrieve or test your sperm, does your doctor specialise in that?

Policies and Procedures

Some clinics have policies about what treatment they will offer. For example, most doctors do not recommend double embryo transfers in IVF. Some cannot do surgical procedures for men and they need to enlist another doctor to help with that. Check whether your clinic can do all the procedures that you want or require.

Other treatments

Does this clinic offer additional and complimentary treatments? Some doctors will not even speak with you about alternative therapy, whereas some doctors offer it as part of their services.

► Do they offer counselling?
► Info nights?
► Support groups?
► Nutritional advice?
► Supplementation advice?

▶ Acupuncture and Chinese medicine?

▶ Yoga?

▶ Day spa?

Instinct

▶ How do you feel about the clinic and the doctor?

▶ Do you feel you are being listened to?

▶ Are your questions being answered properly?

▶ What is your intuition telling you?

Going overseas?

You might consider the option of going overseas for your fertility treatment. That decision really depends upon your specific fertility issues and the treatment you need. You might choose to seek fertility treatment overseas to get a cheaper price or because they have different laws and options available for surrogacy, donor eggs, sperm and embryos. Make sure you still check all the details above and compare prices with local providers, factoring in the additional costs of travelling overseas. Be clear about where your eggs, sperm and embryos would eventually be stored or where your baby would be born. Consider how you will manage the additional stress and uncertainty of travelling for treatment.

The most important thing is that you and your partner are comfortable with your clinic, so don't ignore your instincts. In the end, it is particularly important that the female is happy with the choice. She will interact with the clinic a lot more than you will. Help her do the research, put in your preferences, help her narrow the list down and make the final decision together.

FROM LAURA

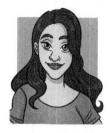

For our own IVF treatment, we chose a doctor who was kind, but direct and honest. We didn't need information to be sugar-coated. We wanted the truth on a plate, with a side of optimism.

One thing we really liked about our fertility doctor was a willingness to try different things after a treatment had been unsuccessful. They say the definition of insanity is trying the same thing over and over, expecting a different result. Some fertility doctors just do the same protocol over and over again and hope for the best. When you first choose a fertility doctor, you don't even consider the idea that your first cycle may not work, but you should. Ask your doctor how they would handle a second attempt if the first one is unsuccessful. It's a great question that could really give some insight into how this doctor would handle a difficult case.

YOUR FIRST APPOINTMENT

Now that you have chosen your fertility specialist, you'll book your first consultation. Most likely you will feel good because you are making progress. You might also feel a little sad to have reached this stage. It's all perfectly normal, there are a lot of conflicting emotions at play.

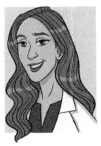

A common worry for anyone facing infertility is the concern that they may not be a parent or they may not have the family they assumed they would.
Coming to terms with the lack of control of family building for the 1 in 8 couples with infertility takes time, processing, and evaluating all options.
- Dr Lora Shahine

You should go to the initial appointment together. Don't leave your partner or baby-making team alone on this one. There will be some appointments that you don't need to attend, but the first appointment is not one of them. Show up as a team, let her know you are in this from the start.

Initially, there is a lot of paperwork. Get on to it straight away, you don't want to be delayed waiting for something to be processed. It seems like there are a lot of forms that you need to fill out, but remember how much paperwork is required to buy a house or a car. This is even more important, it is the paperwork to create a tiny human. Even before your appointment, you can ask the clinic to email the papers to you so you can read through them in advance.

Your first meeting with your doctor can feel like a whirlwind. Go in prepared and have a list of questions written out. We both kept a list of questions for the doctor saved on our phones. We would always have a quick read through before we went into the fertility specialist office, just to make sure we were both on the same page. You pay good money for these short appointments, so you may as well get your money's worth. Some people even like to make an audio recording of the appointment so they can review it afterwards.

It can happen that fertility doctors and nurses will pay little attention to the man and focus more attention on the woman, so you should be prepared for that. It might hurt your feelings or make you feel ignored, however, it is simply a fact that birthing a baby is mostly women's business. Advocate for yourself, speak up. Politely and kindly make sure your questions are answered. Work together with your partner to make sure you both get what you need at the doctor's appointments.

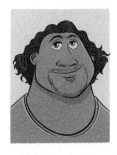

I think the assumption from our IVF clinic was that my wife was the patient and she got all the information and all the feedback forms were sent to her. And I thought, 'Hang on, there are two people in this equation, you have completely ignored me'. I was just staggered that they didn't even send a feedback form to the male partner. **- André**

In all areas of medicine, patients need to be involved in their own care. It would be silly to blindly trust someone else just because they are a medical professional. You should be listened to by your doctor and made to feel that you are active participants in your treatment. They should share your medical information with you openly and listen to your concerns and questions.

Of course, it is important to remember that you need to be a good patient. Fertility clinics deal with lots of people who are experiencing intense emotions and sometimes the staff can cop some unfair treatment. You need to be active in your own health care, but at the same time, you need to be willing to listen and understand what your doctor is saying. Come to your appointments prepared to ask questions and listen to the answers. You may have done extensive research online, but that is just not the same as years and years of medical training and experience.

Some tips for your doctor's appointments:

▶ Expect a lot from your doctor (and find a new doctor if you are not getting what you need).

▶ Be a good patient, be prepared and ask good questions. Be an active participant in your own treatment.

▶ Go to as many appointments with your partner as you can. Be engaged, present and supportive of each other.

▶ Expect that the doctor might be running late. It's just the way it is sometimes!

▶ Keep a list of questions for your fertility specialist. Write them in your phone or in a document that you share with your partner. Whenever you think of something you would like to ask, get into the habit of writing it down immediately. Delete or mark questions once you have been able to ask them.

▶ Record your doctor's appointments. Use your phone (there are even apps designed for recording medical appointments). Or just jot down some notes immediately after or during the appointment – whatever is easiest for you.

▶ Don't be embarrassed. It might be unusual for you to discuss sperm and periods, but for your specialist it is a normal everyday occurrence.

▶ Tell the truth. Your doctor needs the whole truth and nothing but the truth.

▶ Take a few moments during the appointment to take some deep breaths and pause. Make sure you are covering everything you need to talk about. Check in with your partner to ensure that she has been able to ask all her questions too. Incidentally, if you forget to ask something, you can always call or email the clinic to ask later.

QUESTIONS TO ASK YOUR FERTILITY SPECIALIST

Below is a list of potential questions to ask your fertility doctor. You may not need to ask all of them, so you should tailor the list to your needs.

Download this list at www.InfertilityMan.com/MansGuide and you can edit it for your situation.

Diagnosis

▶ What is my diagnosis?
▶ What is my partner's diagnosis?
▶ Is this diagnosis likely to get worse over time, stay the same or improve with treatment?
▶ If our infertility diagnosis is unclear, what tests can we do now to investigate further?

Treatment

▶ Which treatment do you recommend we try first? Why?
▶ Are less invasive or lower tech treatments an option for us?
▶ How soon can we start?
▶ What are the side effects or risks to this treatment?
▶ What are the success rates for couples our age with this treatment?
▶ If this treatment is unsuccessful, what can we try next?
▶ Do you recommend taking a break and skipping a menstrual cycle between treatment cycles? Why do you recommend that?
▶ How many cycles of treatment would you recommend before trying another option?
▶ Does your clinic offer access to donor sperm/eggs/embryos?
▶ In your opinion, how likely is fertility treatment going to be successful for us?

While no doctor can give you an exact answer to this question, considering your personal medical information and age, your doctor's past experiences may allow them to estimate whether you will have an average, below-average, or above-average chance of success.

Lifestyle

- ► Is there anything we can do to improve our chances of success before, during, and after treatment?
- ► What kind of diet do you recommend?
- ► Are there any complementary therapies you recommend?
- ► Are there any supplements you recommend?

AFTER THE APPOINTMENT

Some doctor's appointments you just know are going to be 'big'. Sometimes you will get big news, good or bad, or you may hear something that is difficult to deal with emotionally. Plan that you will need to spend some time with your partner or baby-making team after the appointment, to digest together what was said and make sure you're all ok.

Go to a nice cafe, sit and allow each other time to repeat and think about what you have heard. Do it over a nice cup of coffee or a good meal.

It sometimes helps to stay out in public; it might help you keep your emotions in check. Alternatively, if your partner is upset or if you're feeling upset yourself, head home right away and look after yourselves.

FROM JON

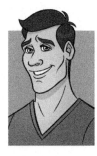

We went to a lot of doctor's appointments together. In a way, it was fun. We always went to one of our favourite cafes afterwards and made it like a date. We did so many back-to-back egg retrievals that we rarely got unexpected news from the doctor, just check-ups and the advice to 'keep going'. We tried to make it a fun experience.

We had two doctors, one for me and one for her. Most often, we went to see the doctor who was focused on the female side of things. On one occasion, we went to see my doctor to talk about my upcoming procedure. He had a different manner. He was super intelligent, very factual, and straight down the line. I thought it was a great appointment. I found the information very useful and the plan we were putting together seemed smart to me.

It wasn't until we got to the elevator on the way out of the building that I even realised that this appointment had not felt so good to Laura. As soon as the doors closed, she quietly burst into tears. I racked my brain to think of what could have upset her? I couldn't see anything in what the doctor had said that would be worth being worried about.

I tried to reason with her. "I thought that was a good appointment. I thought everything he said made sense. I thought that we have a good plan in place."

This only made her cry more. It felt like we were arguing. I realised that reasoning with her probably wasn't the best strategy. Something about that appointment upset her, and it didn't really matter what it was. It turned out that it wasn't really about the doctor, it was just the heavy load of months of fertility treatment. This was just the straw that broke the camel's back.

In the end, there was only one thing to do. I gave her a long hug and just let her cry for a little while. When she was finished, I took her home and tucked her up in bed. She went to sleep and I went to work. That is just how infertility is sometimes.

TIME FOR TESTS

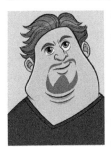

It's weird; I always had a feeling that I was infertile. I've always thought it, since I was a kid. When my Mrs and I started trying, they ran all the tests under the sun on her and they never even thought about testing me. When they did eventually test me, the result came back as zero sperm. It was a big eye opener, it woke me up, it changed my life… it changed our lives. **- Ben**

Ensure that your doctor does a full analysis of both of you. Sometimes, men are channelled from their GP and sent straight to a doctor in an IVF clinic who doesn't specialise in the male reproductive system. Sometimes these doctors can focus all their attention on the female. It is so important that both the male and the female are checked out; too often couples spend months and even years not understanding their own infertility because the man has not had adequate testing.

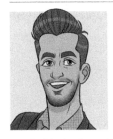

90% of people who come to me for an initial consultation with fertility issues assume the problem is with the female. I met with a lovely couple that were having trouble getting pregnant. They had seen their general practitioner and the man had already done two semen analyses, both of which were vastly abnormal. The GP's advice was, 'Oh well, you probably had a cold or something which has affected your sperm sample and reduced the number of sperm. Do another test in 3 months.'

The next sperm sample was still abnormal, but the GP said not to worry about it. He suggested they see a specialist just to get some reassurance. I saw the results of the sperm tests and told them they had significant male factor infertility. The sample had 1 million sperm per millilitre, which is not normal and is not explained by a transient illness. I asked if he had even been unwell lately and he said no. I told them they needed to see an IVF specialist and they were floored. It really took a while for them to process it. People think that infertility is just a female issue… and it's not. **- Dr Scott Shemer**

For Males...

Fertility testing for males can be divided into two categories; tests for the man and tests for the sperm. Only when both have been examined thoroughly can the doctor reach a full diagnosis.

Testing for the Man

▶ Clinical History. The doctor should get a full picture of his medical history. What is his pregnancy history? Did he experience anything in his past that might be contributing to his infertility? Did he have mumps as a child? An undescended testicle? Cancer and chemotherapy? A rugby injury that might have damaged his testicles? Does he take any medication now that might be affecting his sperm? Any previous surgeries that might be relevant? Has he been exposed to chemicals or toxins that might cause issues? Is he a smoker?

▶ Clinical Examination. The doctor should physically examine the testicles, checking for things like varicoceles or other abnormalities. They might also perform a scrotal ultrasound. This test uses high-frequency sound waves to look at the testicles and supporting structures.

▶ Blood Tests. Standard screening tests need only include – Follicle Stimulating Hormone, Luteinising Hormone, Testosterone and a semen analysis. If any of these show a problem then more tests may be needed: Prolactin, Oestradiol, Thyroid Levels and an Ultrasound of testicles. If IVF is needed, other blood tests will need to be done for Sexually Transmitted Diseases, for example Syphilis, Chlamydia, Gonorrhoea, HIV, Hepatitis B and Hepatitis C.

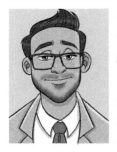 *It is just so important to appreciate that in 50% of couples who cannot conceive, a male factor is at least partially to blame. Therefore, the guy does need to be assessed thoroughly. This includes a full and detailed medical history and very importantly, a physical examination. There are multiple causes as to why men may have problems with fertility. Some of these can be assessed through talking to the patient but others are revealed only when you are examined. If you are assessed by a doctor who only gives you a cup to produce a semen sample, then perhaps you should ask them for a full examination.*

*Some causes of male infertility, when treated, can actually end up fixing the problem and allowing the couple to conceive naturally. A varicocele (a clump of varicose veins above the testicle) may be such a cause. It is best detected during a physical examination. Removal of a varicocele (especially bigger ones) has been shown to improve sperm counts and natural pregnancy. Furthermore, if IVF ends up being needed, when the varicocele is removed the success rates may be improved. Therefore it is also important that your specialist check for varicoceles during the assessment. - **Dr Darren Katz**

Testing for Sperm

A Semen Analysis will check
► Sperm count, the number of sperm per millilitre
► Motility (the sperm's ability to move)
► Morphology (the sperm's size and shape)
► Volume and consistency of the ejaculated sample.

Sperm testing should also look at pH levels, antisperm antibodies and DNA fragmentation.

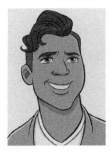

We started with the female testing to make sure that everything was working with her and that all checked out. So the next step was to check with me and I assumed I would be ok. It was kind of a shock when the nurse told me I had zero sperm. You're kind of in denial. I took the sperm test two more times. When they both came back with zero, I started to believe that it was true. **- José**

How to Give a Sperm Sample

Let's be honest, these tests have a reputation for being uncomfortable and embarrassing. However, it really doesn't have to be and your partner or baby-making team is counting on you to get it done.

Have a think about how you can make yourself more comfortable in order to produce your sample. Some clinics require you to do it on their premises, some allow you to produce the sample at home and bring it in soon afterwards.

FROM JON

Before going to give my sperm samples, I had the craziest thoughts...

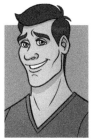

- ▶ *How much porn could there possibly be?*
- ▶ *What options will I have?*
- ▶ *Will they provide lubricant?*
- ▶ *Will it be clean?*
- ▶ *Will anyone interrupt me? I must make sure I lock the door!*

The process was relatively painless and somewhat unexciting. I was told I could do it at home and bring it in to the clinic within 30 minutes or I could book an appointment at the facility. I booked at the clinic and on my arrival was ushered to a room with nothing more than a chair, table and tissues. I was given a sample cup in a plastic bag and I was to drop it in the tray on the way out. There was no need to meet with anyone after the job was done.

Many clinics now expect that men will provide their own entertainment on their own phone. With a little imagination, you can pull up anything you need in order to get the job done.

The results went to my GP and my fertility specialist. The Result? No sperm at all in my ejaculate.

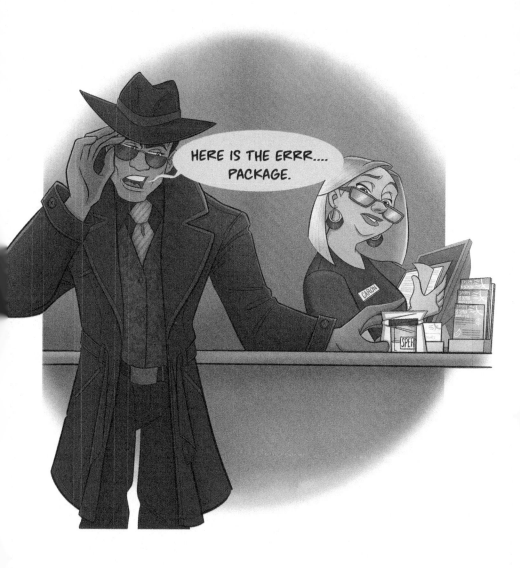

How to get the most out of your Semen Test.

▶ Don't ejaculate for at least two days before giving your sample, but make sure you have ejaculated in the previous ten days. Samples produced after two days of abstinence have the highest possible concentration of good-looking, strong swimming sperm.

▶ Don't drink alcohol in the few days before providing your sample.

▶ Bring your own adult entertainment or imagine your partner.

▶ Wash your hands and penis before you start.

▶ Set yourself up right with everything you need close by and take the lid off the cup.

▶ Don't use any lubricant, cream or saliva.

▶ Try to collect the first part of the ejaculate as it is thought to contain the most sperm.

▶ Avoid spilling any of your sample. If you do spill, don't try to scrape it off what is likely a contaminated surface.

▶ If you are producing your sample at home instead of at the clinic, make sure you get it there as quickly as possible in less than an hour.

▶ If you are transporting it, keep the sample at body temperature by putting it in your pocket.

Check these points with your doctor to make sure you are providing the sample within their recommendations.

Be aware that recent illness can affect the results of your semen analysis.

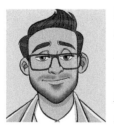

If a patient comes to me and they have a poor sperm count, I ask them if they have been unwell in the lead up to their test. Sperm take around two to three months to go from an immature cell into a mature sperm and if over that journey the man has been unwell, it may affect his sperm count. **- Dr Darren Katz**

Finally, don't be embarrassed. These doctors and nurses see this every single day. They are not worried by it, so why should you be? Be proud of yourself that you are taking such active steps to solving the puzzle that is your fertility.

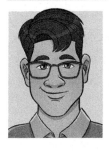

It's the things you go through when you're in this struggle, you have those feelings of not being good enough. I remember after the first two cycles I said to our fertility specialist, 'What do you need me to do? I don't care, I'll take every test, whatever procedure is required, anything.' I'm not proud, if something is wrong, I want to know. I don't want to put my wife through hell because I am too stubborn or proud to see if I am a contributing factor. - Caleb

For Females...

Below is a list of some common tests, some are for fertility and some are good to do before any pregnancy. Your doctor will test these things to help them reach a diagnosis and to get an idea of how she may respond to fertility medications.

► Blood tests, Iron, Vitamin D, Vitamin B12, Zinc and Homocysteine, etc.
► Hormone Levels, such as, Oestrogen, Follicle Stimulating Hormone, Luteinising Hormone, Prolactin, Oestradiol, Progesterone and Thyroid Levels.
► Pre-pregnancy checks such as Folate levels, Human T-lymphotropic virus, Varicella (chickenpox), Rubella (German Measles), Parvovirus & Cytomegalovirus, Ureaplasma and Mycoplasma, and Cystic Fibrosis.
► Sexually Transmitted Diseases, for example Syphilis, Chlamydia, Gonorrhoea, HIV, Hepatitis B and Hepatitis C.

Anti-Müllerian hormone (AMH) is a hormone secreted by cells in the developing egg sacs (follicles). Measuring the level of this hormone in her blood can give an indication of her egg reserve. If the number is low, then she may have lowered egg reserve.

It is important to remember that women with a low ovarian reserve and women with a high ovarian reserve fall pregnant naturally at the same rate. This is because women in both groups ovulate one egg per month and one egg equals one baby (two in the case of identical twins, or more for multiple births). AMH doesn't indicate the quality of the eggs.

AMH is a useful tool for predicting how well she may respond to IVF, and give an idea of the likely egg number that will be retrieved from an egg retrieval.

This is a very general test and can't tell you everything about her fertility, but it is a great place to start. Don't freak out if the result is not what you expected, her AMH number is only one indicator of your chance to have a baby. It is always better to know what is going on than to be in the dark.

Follicle stimulating hormone (FSH) is produced by the pituitary gland in the brain. This hormone controls the menstrual cycle and stimulates the ovaries to produce eggs. If the result of her blood test shows elevated FSH (a high number), it suggests that the brain is having to produce more follicle stimulating hormone to work the ovaries harder to produce the egg each month indicating that her ovaries are not working at an optimal level or that she is approaching menopause.

Pelvic Ultrasound

Female fertility testing usually includes a pelvic ultrasound to check what is happening inside the uterus. The doctor will look at the ovaries as well, where they can see how many follicles, with eggs potentially inside, your partner is producing each month. They should also look at the fallopian tubes to rule out any blockages.

Before she has this examination, ask her how she feels about it. Find out whether she would like you to come into the room with her for moral support, or if she would prefer to go in alone for more privacy. As an extra 'heads up', be aware that women who have experienced sexual assault might find these examinations especially challenging.

FROM LAURA

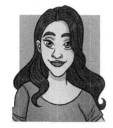

When I went for my first ultrasound, I thought it would be like on TV where they put some gel on your tummy and you sit up and look excitedly at the screen. It was not at all like that. It was an internal scan, so they put a condom and some lubricant on a pointy wand and gently put it up inside the vagina.

It is a little undignified, but it doesn't hurt. It can definitely be uncomfortable, but you will get used to it. If you go on to have fertility treatment, you will have many, many more of these internal scans.

BABY-MAKING MEET UP

Knowledge is power, but execution – actually doing something is even more powerful. Wherever you are on your baby-making journey, now is the time to take action.

Hopefully, things will go well and you will solve this challenge quickly. However oftentimes, these things take far longer than you expect them to, especially if you end up needing fertility treatment, so it's best to get started right away.

With your partner or Baby-Making Team:

► Make an appointment with your doctor for fertility testing.
► Discuss what is important to you when choosing a fertility specialist.
► Share with your partner any relevant details about your sexual and medical history, including any past pregnancies. It is better to share this information for the first time in private rather than in a doctor's office.
► Discuss with each other any concerns you may have about the testing process.
► Discuss how you can support each other.
   ► Would you like your partner to come to your appointment with you?
   ► Would your partner prefer you to be in the room for their pelvic exam, or would they prefer some privacy?

See the Baby-Making Meet Up videos and download a workbook at www.InfertilityMan.com/MansGuide

EXPECTATION VERSUS REALITY

Why is infertility such a challenging experience?
Why does it make people feel sad and affect their mental health?

Everyone has some idea of how they expect that their life will turn out. We base these expectations on what we hoped for when we were younger and what we see people around us having (even if what we see isn't an accurate representation of how happy they truly are).

This is particularly so for the dream of having children. We spend our early lives seeing adults seemingly getting pregnant easily and we imagine that this will one day happen for us. We expect our bodies will do what they are 'supposed' to do and produce our children.

But what if they don't?
The equation for happiness is when our expectations equal our reality. We assume we will feel satisfied when we get the outcome that we were hoping for (it may only last for a moment before we are lusting after the next thing, but that is another story!)

When we don't get what we expect or what we think we deserve, that's when we feel disappointed and unhappy. When we compare ourselves with others and notice what they have that we don't, we feel cheated, and that life is unfair.

Life is inherently unfair. Infertility is particularly unfair. Unfortunately, there is not a lot we can do about that.
So how can we be content and even happy while life is being so unfair?

When you aren't 'loving what is', you have two choices: you can either change your expectations or you can change your reality.

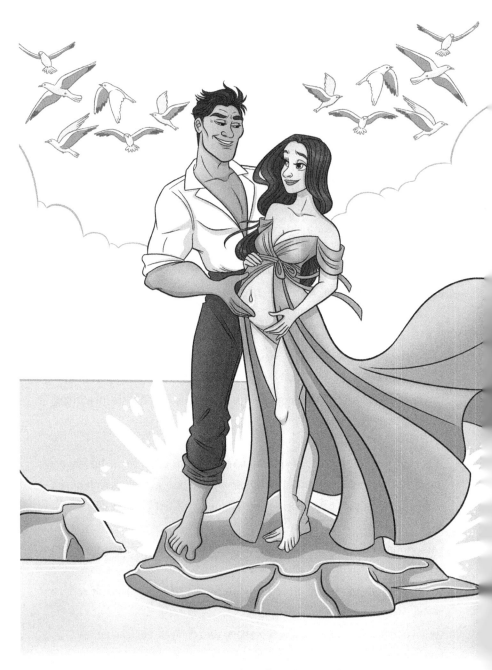

#EXPECTATION

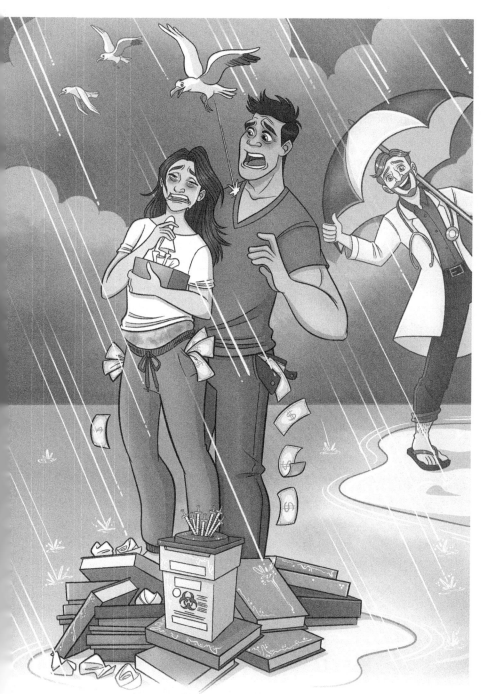

#REALITY

Fertility treatment is an attempt to change your reality. You're hoping to make your situation in the real world different from what it is. There are many moments as you are progressing through your fertility treatment when you will have high expectations and the reality will not be what you are hoping for. These are the moments that could make you or your partner emotional, as it is very disappointing.

This is so challenging and, of course, sometimes it's ok to allow yourself to feel negative emotions – infertility is hard! Unfortunately, trying to conceive can last for a long time, and feeling negative emotions for such a long time could seriously affect your mental health.

Our expectations can get the better of us when we expect more than what is realistic. The other alternative is to alter your expectations to meet your reality. Staying happy during fertility treatment is the most delicate balance of being hopeful, but staying reasonable and flexible in your expectations.

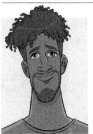

*The doctor said, 'I think two cycles is all it is going to take. We just need to find a good quality embryo.' But when we were two cycles in and nothing had happened, the doctor gave us a completely new set of expectations. Instead of expecting after one or two cycles that we would be pregnant, he told us that on any IVF cycle we would have about a 10% chance of success. We should expect to do up to 10 cycles before we would be successful. So that was pretty tough. - **Lamar**

The antidote to expectations that don't match your reality is gratitude and appreciation. What can you be grateful for in your life, even if it's something small?

We have seen some people doing infertility treatment who are super happy with just one mature egg retrieved and others who are dismayed at 'only fifteen' mature eggs.

On your first IVF cycle you might be bitterly disappointed to create only four embryos, but on your sixth IVF cycle you might be delighted to create two.

It's all a matter of perspective. You must find a way to look after your mental health to have the endurance to continue through this difficult period of your life. We want you to be able to endure until you reach an outcome that you can live with happily.

With your partner or your Baby-Making team, consistently seek out things to be grateful for, even if they are small. Allow yourself time to grieve and then be grateful for every discovery, every egg, sperm, embryo, anything you learn that could help you move forward. Actively celebrate the small wins. Come up with cute ways to acknowledge any little thing that goes well. Appreciate each other and any access you have to this potentially life creating medical technology. While it is unrealistic to expect to be totally happy throughout your infertility experience, actively taking steps to be grateful and protect your mental health will make you more resilient for the journey ahead.

DIAGNOSIS

Being diagnosed with a medical condition can be confusing and a real shock. Receiving the news that your infertility is unexplainable can be equally stressful. To learn that something is standing in your way to conceiving a baby can be overwhelming. It can bring up feelings of disappointment, sadness, and fear. It might cause you to feel guilt for choices you made in the past. It can make you feel regret for not having babies earlier and grief for the babies you think you'll never have.

Some men refuse to accept the news and their denial makes them reluctant and slow to seek treatment options. Some men give up all hope and suggest their partner wouldn't want to be with a man who could never get them pregnant, creating relationship issues. Some men jump straight to 'problem-solving mode', making rash decisions and they miss the chance to fully process what's happening.

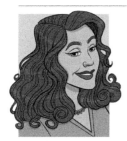 *Men often don't handle an infertility diagnosis very well. For many, it impacts their sense of masculinity and they can feel like they are letting their partner down. And then if the partner has to go through fertility treatment with the injections and everything else, I think some men feel very guilty about that. There is not enough support for men going through fertility treatment. - Dr Lynn Burmeister*

This is a moment when it is really important to connect with your partner (or your baby-making team). Their response might be different from yours, so take time to listen and understand. While a situation like this may initially put strain on your relationship, it is possible to come through this even more united than before. Give them and yourself time and space to feel your reaction. This really sucks. Seek support. Be kind to yourself.

This news might be unexpected or it might be confirmation of a long-held suspicion that something wasn't right. Either way, getting a diagnosis is a positive step (even a diagnosis of unexplained infertility). This is the start of your baby-making journey, not the end. The initial diagnosis is a puzzle to be solved, and if you want to be a parent, you will find a way, even if it is not the way you originally thought it would happen. Your path may not be as you first expected, but be proud of yourself for taking the first steps.

What is Infertility?

The World Health Organisation got together to determine the definition of infertility and here is what they came up with:

Infertility: a disease of the reproductive system defined by the failure to achieve a clinical pregnancy after 12 months or more of regular unprotected sexual intercourse or due to an impairment of a person's capacity to reproduce either as an individual or with his/her partner.

Pretty vague, huh? Basically, anyone who hasn't been able to get pregnant in the natural way is considered infertile. Welcome to the club! It is not a club that anyone ever chooses to be part of (yet there are some pretty cool people in this club, as you will see).

At least one in eight couples need specialist help for infertility at some time in their lives. When one partner has a fertility challenge, then the other person is also affected - remember you don't need to have a diagnosed medical issue yourself to experience infertility with your partner.

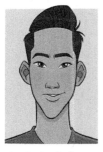 *Infertility invades every part of your life. On a personal level, you have to confront the fact that you might not have a family. It affects you financially, as you try to save to fund the treatment. We had family fallouts because we couldn't see newborn nieces and nephews – we just couldn't be around babies. We changed jobs because time off with certain employers was difficult. I don't think there was any part of our life before that was still there by the end. It strips just about everything away.* **- James**

CAUSES OF INFERTILITY

The results from your fertility testing will place you and your partner
in one of four categories.

► Male Factor Infertility (you are the one who has fertility challenges)
►· Female Factor Infertility (she is the one who has fertility challenges)
► Both Male and Female Factor Infertility (both of you have fertility
   challenges)
► Unexplained Fertility (the tests did not show clear evidence of either of
   you having fertility challenges)

Male Factor Infertility: It can be difficult to hear that your body is the
reason that you are having trouble conceiving naturally. If you receive this
diagnosis, it is important to remember that infertility is nobody's fault.
If you could easily change your situation, you certainly would.

To be able to get a woman pregnant naturally, a number of things must
function optimally.

► You need to produce healthy sperm in the correct shape and size
► Sperm have to be carried in the semen
► There needs to be enough sperm in the semen
► Sperm must be functional and able to move
► You have to be able to perform sex
► Your sperm have to be able to form healthy embryos

Male factor infertility can be due to low sperm production, abnormal sperm
function or blockages that prevent the delivery of sperm. Injuries, illnesses,
chronic health problems, lifestyle choices and other factors can play a role in
causing male infertility.

If male factor infertility is indeed the problem, then you may need to
reassess which doctor you choose to treat you. Ensure that your fertility
specialist has additional training and expertise in male factor infertility or
you might opt for a urologist with skills in that area.

FROM JON

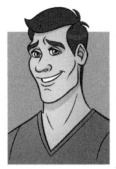

In our case, we soon learned that a regular fertility doctor might not be suitably experienced to manage my male factor infertility. As a result of my testicular cancer and having no sperm in my ejaculate, I required a procedure called a microTESE to see if sperm could be collected directly from my one testicle. The fertility specialists we saw early on offered to do less precise testicular biopsies, but that was just not going to cut it in my case. We learned that there were only a few doctors in our city who were able to perform the microTESE procedure, and one of them was particularly well qualified. He was a urologist who did not do assisted reproductive procedures for females, so we ended up with two separate clinics, one for Laura and one for me. It took a bit of organising to get the schedules of both doctors aligned, but we are so glad that we had two top specialists, one in male factor and one in female factor infertility.

Here is a list of some of the common male infertility causes, with a description in simple language.

Medical Factors

▶ **Problems with sexual intercourse**
This can include difficulty getting or maintaining an erection sufficient for sex or premature ejaculation (otherwise known as erectile dysfunction). Perhaps there are psychological or relationship problems that interfere with sex.

▶ **Ejaculation issues**
In some guys, semen enters the bladder during orgasm instead of coming out the penis. Spinal cord injuries or certain diseases sometimes make it difficult or impossible for some men to ejaculate semen, even though they may still produce sperm.

▶ Hormone imbalances

The hormones might be out of balance from a disorder in the testicles or perhaps something in the brain that is not working correctly. Testosterone, oestrogen, luteinising hormone and follicle stimulating hormone must be in balance for sperm production.

▶ Infection

Some infections can interfere with sperm production or sperm health. An infection might cause scarring, which may block where the sperm are trying to get out. This can be caused by inflammation or some sexually transmitted diseases.

▶ Sperm Antibodies

These are immune system cells that mistakenly identify sperm as harmful invaders and attempt to eliminate them.

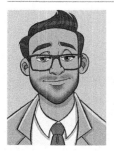

*If patients have a high degree of sperm antibodies and are not conceiving naturally, then IVF is a good solution to that problem. People talk about giving steroids and things like that to try to overcome sperm antibodies, but the literature and the science behind that is poor and the side effect profile is high. If a patient comes to me with sperm antibodies, and there is no other reversible cause found or no other way to improve their fertility potential, I direct them to an IVF specialist. - **Dr Darren Katz**

▶ Tumours

Cancers and non-malignant (not cancerous) tumours can affect male fertility.

▶ Undescended testicles

In some men, one or both of the testicles don't descend from the abdomen into the sac where they are supposed to live. If a man has had this condition, he is more likely to have fertility issues.

► *Defects of tubules that transport sperm.*

Sperm travels through several tubes before it reaches its final destination. These tubes can be blocked for lots of different reasons, like prior infections, trauma, injury or abnormal development.

► *Chromosome defects*

Genetic syndromes can cause abnormal development of the male reproductive organs. Disorders that can affect fertility include cystic fibrosis, Kallmann syndrome, Kartagener syndrome and Klinefelter syndrome.

► *Celiac/Coeliac disease*

This is a digestive disorder caused by sensitivity to gluten, and it can affect male fertility.

► *Certain medications*

Some medications can affect sperm production and affect male fertility like testosterone replacement therapy, steroids or chemotherapy.

► *Prior Surgeries*

Previous surgeries can prevent men from having sperm in their ejaculate. If a man has had a vasectomy, scrotal or testicular surgery, a hernia repair or surgery performed for testicular and rectal cancers, it may affect his fertility.

► *Varicocele*

A varicocele is a swelling of the veins that send blood to and from the testicle. Sometimes they grow too big and tangle which can make the testicle heat up and impair sperm function. This can often be fixed with surgery, which in turn can improve sperm quality, numbers and function.

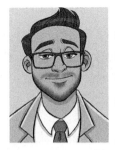

The optimal temperature to make sperm is about 2 to 3 degrees below core body temperature. That is why the testicles hang lower when it's hot and they are closer to the body when it's cool - this helps to create the perfect environment for producing sperm.

The testicle is a fragile organ and many things can cause it to not function well. A varicocele is essentially varicose veins sitting above the testicle. It's quite common, about 15% of men have a varicocele and most of the time it doesn't cause any problems. However, in some men, it can cause issues with the sperm, such as DNA fragmentation and difficulty conceiving. Varicoceles carry the blood from the testicles back into the body and if they are too large or there is a problem with them, then there is too much heat going on all the time.

The testicles can't get to that optimal temperature to make sperm. Another theory is that varicoceles release free radicals, which can cause problems with the DNA. Each patient presenting with a varicocele must be considered individually. I look at several things:

- The size of the varicocele: smaller ones may be less important, bigger ones may cause more difficulties.
- The size of the testicles, often you can see a bit of shrinkage.
- The semen analysis, paying attention to certain patterns.
- DNA Fragmentation.

Surgery to correct the varicocele could be helpful, as removing them can improve the environment in which the sperm are made. I've taken out varicoceles in men who were deemed to be infertile and they have gone on to have children. Many studies show that in patients who have low sperm count, if you remove a varicocele, it can increase. What is less well known is that removing varicoceles can also improve IVF outcomes.

A lot of people think that the sperm is there only to go into the egg and make an embryo. In fact, we know that the quality of the sperm makes a difference all the way through pregnancy, during the first, second and even up to the third trimester. A man's varicocele can be a factor in why couples are having recurring early miscarriages, so it is important that the man is checked. - **Dr Darren Katz**

Environmental Factors

Believe it or not, the environment that your testicles are exposed to can affect your fertility. Elements such as heat, toxins and chemicals can reduce sperm production, quality or function.

▶ *Overheating*
Warm temperatures can impair sperm production and function. Although studies are inconclusive, frequent use of saunas or hot tubs may temporarily reduce your sperm count. Sitting for long periods with your testes tucked up too warm, wearing tight underwear or sitting with a laptop computer on your lap for long stretches of time may increase the temperature in your scrotum and reduce sperm production.

▶ *Industrial chemicals*
Low sperm counts may be caused by extended exposure to pesticides, herbicides, organic solvents, painting materials, benzenes, toluene, xylene and lead.

▶ *Radiation or x-rays*
Exposure to radiation can reduce sperm production, although it usually returns to normal eventually. High doses could cause a permanent reduction in sperm count.

Lifestyle and Health Factors

More and more research is showing that how you live your life, how healthy you are physically and emotionally can affect your fertility.

▶ *Drug use*
Anabolic steroids can cause the testicles to shrink and sperm production to decrease. Cocaine, marijuana and other recreational drugs may reduce the number and quality of sperm.

▶ *Alcohol use*

Drinking alcohol may lower testosterone levels, decrease sperm production and cause erectile dysfunction. Liver disease caused by excessive drinking may also lead to fertility issues.

▶ *Smoking*

Among all the many other health issues that smoking causes, fertility is also affected. Second-hand smoke may cause problems too. Men who ingest smoke may have a lower sperm count than those who don't.

▶ *Stress*

Stress can interfere with hormones needed to produce sperm. Prolonged emotional stress may affect sperm count.

▶ *Depression*

Depression can cause sexual dysfunction like reduced libido, erectile dysfunction or issues with ejaculation.

▶ *Weight*

Obesity or being very underweight can impact fertility in several ways, either directly on the sperm or on the hormones that can affect male fertility.

These are just some of the issues that might be highlighted by your fertility tests. Make sure you get your doctor to explain your diagnosis in a way that you can understand.

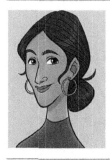

We have no idea why my hubby has no sperm. He used to play lacrosse professionally as a goalie in Canada for many years, so it could be due to trauma to his testicles from being hit by the ball. He has low testosterone and high FSH, which indicates there's a problem somewhere. But you would never think it if you saw him. He's 6'4" and 105kg of muscle! - **Louise**

LET'S TALK ABOUT SPERM

What are the factors that determine healthy sperm? It comes down to three main qualities.

1. *Quantity* (volume). If you have 15 million or more for every millilitre of semen, that would be classed as a healthy sperm count.
2. *Movement* (motility). Just like some guys on the dance floor, not every sperm moves efficiently, effectively or even at all.
3. *Shape* (morphology). A rounded head with a long and strong tail is usually what a healthy sperm would look like.

Azoospermia

Azoospermia is the complete absence of sperm in the semen.
There are two types of azoospermia: obstructive and non-obstructive.

Obstructive
If there is some obstacle in the way, a man may be producing sperm normally but it just can't get from the testicles into the ejaculate. There may be some issue with the vas deferens, which is the tube that transports the sperm to the penis. It may be blocked due to infection, injury, or vasectomy.

Non-obstructive
The testicles may produce little or no sperm at all, perhaps due to genetic conditions like Klinefelter syndrome or a previous condition like mumps. Sometimes small amounts of sperm can be found in these men and used to create embryos using ICSI technology (when the sperm is injected into the egg using a needle so they don't have to swim on their own).
In some men, the pituitary gland is non-functioning, so even though they have the tools they need to make sperm, they just don't. Sometimes, hormone injections can jump start sperm production to give these men a shot at having their own biological children.

Oligozoospermia – Low Sperm Count

This tongue twister refers to low sperm count, meaning there are less sperm per sample than the established norm. This does not necessarily mean that conception is impossible, though medical help may be necessary.

Asthenozoospermia – Poor Motility

If the doctor throws this word around, then the sperm are not swimming properly, which means they may not find the egg or be strong enough to get to the egg.

Hypospermia – Low Semen Volume

This refers to a below average amount of semen delivered with each ejaculation. It does not necessarily affect the sperm count.

Teratozoospermia – Atypical Morphology/Shape

The size and shape of the majority of sperm are abnormal, for example, they may have misshaped heads or multiple tails.

Sperm DNA Fragmentation and Damage

Sperm DNA fragmentation occurs when there is a change in the bases or a physical break in one or both of the DNA strands of the chromosomes contained within the sperm. DNA fragmentation is measured by a semen analysis.

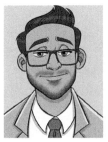

*All sperm has some degree of DNA fragmentation. As it passes through the parts of the testicle and the penis, the overall sperm fragmentation increases. If a patient has sperm seen in their ejaculate and the DNA fragmentation is very high, then taking sperm directly out of the testicle through surgery can result in better outcomes. Many couples ask me if they have a high DNA fragmentation level does that mean that, if they have children, the children will have problems with their DNA? The answer to this is no. DNA fragmentation is normal, but if patient has a high level of DNA fragmentation it may be more difficult to conceive. However, it does not mean that the patient's child will have genetic issues. This is important to clarify. - **Dr Darren Katz**

Receiving Your Fertility Report Card

It is important to keep a copy of your tests results. You might not understand them very well at the start, but over time you will become very good at reading your results. Over time, you may notice patterns and observe your results improving or deteriorating.

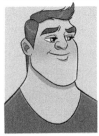

*When it turned out that I had azoospermia, I kind of went into shock and into denial. I was kind of grieving, I was pretty sad, you know? I cried a lot and I was like, 'Man, what is happening?' We both cried a lot. We didn't really know what the next step was. - **Pete**

The results of your sperm test are a medical diagnosis. It does not define you as a person. There is nothing personal here, just another problem to solve. This is an opportunity to show integrity, bravery, and vulnerability.

Your diagnosis is just the beginning of your infertility journey. The good news is, in some cases, sperm quality can be improved. You can change your lifestyle to increase your chance of producing better sperm in the future. In some cases, sperm can be retrieved directly from the testicles through surgery and injected directly into the eggs during IVF. Your doctor will advise you of the next steps.

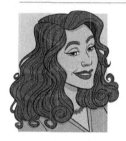

Poor quality sperm can still create good quality embryos. The egg can 'fix up' the damage in sperm. If it is a good egg, it can repair the sperm.

- Dr Lynn Burmeister

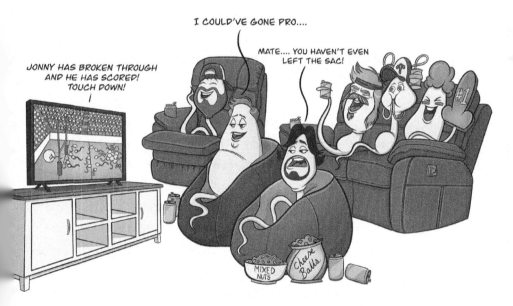

FROM JON

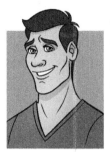

Ever since I became sexually active, I would hear stories about guys accidentally getting someone pregnant at a young age. It never happened to me when I was younger and I was quite relieved about that.

I guess with my diagnosis, I now know why. It clearly wasn't just down to dumb luck.

Knowing all I know today, so many things line up to explain where I am right now. I had an undescended testicle as a baby. Testicular torsion required emergency surgery at York Children's Hospital in Scotland when I was about 18 months old. Apparently, men who have experienced undescended testicles have an increased risk of testicular cancer.

Throughout my teens, I had issues with Gynaecomastia, when males develop breast tissue because of an imbalanced ratio of oestrogen and androgen activity. I've always been unusually tall, and I grew very fast, which had some uncomfortable side effects such as growing pains. These issues in my early life potentially led to my testicular cancer as an adult.

It's highly likely that I have never had any sperm in my ejaculate, therefore I couldn't have gotten anyone pregnant if I tried. If I had known that as I was growing up, I might have felt differently about my relationships and my future.

When I was diagnosed with cancer, I thought my doctor told me I couldn't ever have kids (a mistake on my part). I suppose I heard what I could process at that time.

Later, a sperm test showed I had no sperm in my ejaculate. In my past relationships, my partners never seemed to want to have kids. I decided that supporting other people's kids was where my energies needed to go, so I began mentoring young people and coaching them in sport and things like that. If I couldn't have my own, then I would just look after everyone else's and give them back afterwards. Even before I truly investigated my infertility, I had resigned myself to a childless life, and I was ok with that. Looking back, I realise I had simply turned my attention away from the issue as a kind of denial, rather than facing it head on.

Then I met Laura and on our first date we were talking about children and she asked if I wanted kids. I emphatically replied, "Yes! But unfortunately, I can't have my own children." I don't think she realised how powerful her next question was, because it set me off on a hunt for answers.

All she asked was, "Is that really true? Have you had it properly tested lately?"

I thought I was infertile, I believed the doctor many years ago had told me I could never have kids. However, when I really thought about it, I think now that what he said was "You will have to look at other ways to have children."

Remembering this differently, I thought it wouldn't hurt to get tested and explore a little deeper. Even though Laura and I had only known each other for a few weeks, off I went and found a doctor, then a reproductive specialist.

I looked into the possibility that I might have been producing sperm, but it was not getting out. It was quite the change in my life when a definite 'no' on kids became a 'possible maybe'. Any hope is better than no hope at all.

Female Factor Infertility: This may be hard on your partner. She may feel some very unwelcome negative feelings about her diagnosis, fear about the future and maybe even that she has let you down. Connect with her, show her affection, and give her a lot of reassurance that a diagnosis like this doesn't define her as a person.

There are many reasons for female infertility. It could be caused by autoimmune diseases or hormone issues such as PCOS (Polycystic ovarian syndrome). Structural issues like fibroids, polyps, blocked or missing fallopian tubes, endometriosis or genetic conditions like cystic fibrosis or Turner syndrome. Egg quality declines with age, so your partner's age may be the cause of your infertility. There are many books, websites and resources about female factor infertility, so seek out information to help you understand the diagnosis.

Both Male and Female Factor Infertility: Some couples find themselves in the category of having both male and female factor infertility. This can be challenging, but not insurmountable. It will be important to get a good understanding of the issues on both sides so that you can see how they might impact each other. You may process your separate diagnoses differently, so be kind to each other during this time.

Unexplained Infertility: When the medical tests have been done, and the doctors still can not find a cause for your infertility, it is called unexplained infertility or idiopathic infertility. This can be challenging on a number of levels. What do you do next when medical science comes back to you, shrugs its shoulders and says, "I dunno?"

In a way, it is good because at least you don't have a confirmed medical condition. In another way, it sucks! Because… what do you do next?

When the doctor looks at your tests and says "Good news, we found nothing wrong with you" they should instead say "Bad news, we found nothing wrong with you ... we have no clue! So I'm going to sign you up for more uncomfortable tests, a few years of emotional distress on a roller coaster that you never know if it is going to end, financial stress and more heartbreak than you think you can bear. Sound good?"

This is the reason that unexplained infertility is a challenge. It's hard to fix a problem if you don't know what the problem is. Make sure your doctor explains everything to you to help you understand. While it can be helpful to look to online resources to learn more about your diagnosis, be careful not to fall down an internet rabbit hole. You must make really conscious choices right now to protect your mental health.

Unexplained infertility can be difficult to solve, but there is always more to discover. Work with your doctor to establish what further tests and examinations could shed some light on what is preventing you from getting pregnant. With time, you may find an explanation for your unexplained infertility.

Many couples with unexplained infertility never figure out what is wrong. They simply proceed with fertility treatment and hopefully get pregnant.

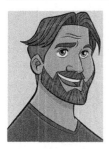 *After only 6 months of trying to conceive naturally we thought, 'let's not f*** around, something is not working, let's go and check it out.' On paper, we were ideal candidates for IVF. We were both reasonably young; we had good egg count, good mature, healthy eggs, and I had no problem with my sperm. Our problem was attrition. In the first round we got 16 eggs, 10 fertilised naturally.*

*On Day 3, they called us to tell us that 10 out of 10 were still growing. We were like, 'Oh my goodness, this is unbelievable, we're going to smash this.' Day 5 came around and we went in for our first transfer. As soon as I saw the embryologist's face, I thought 'Something is not right'. She said, 'Look, we do have one to transfer, the others are looking a bit slow.' Then, all the remaining embryos just died. The embryologist said she had never seen attrition like it. And so did the one we put back, that was an unsuccessful transfer. So began our three and a half years of struggle with unexplained infertility. The problem that still haunts us, even now that we have had success, is that there was never a reason given, there was never anything you could put a finger on. The really hard thing for us was just never having an answer. - **Josh***

Primary or Secondary Infertility?

Fertility patients are divided into two more categories: primary and secondary infertility. If you have never carried pregnancy through to a live birth, then you fall into the primary infertility group. Secondary infertility is the inability to conceive a child or carry a pregnancy to full term after previously giving birth without help from fertility medications or treatments, like in vitro fertilization.

WHOSE FAULT IS IT?

Before we go any further, it's important to acknowledge that infertility is nobody's 'fault'. It really doesn't matter who has the body that is not performing exactly as it is supposed to, you are in this together.

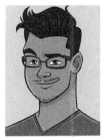

We had a conversation where she said 'leave me now, while you still have a chance to find someone who can get pregnant and have a child with you.' And I was like, 'You're my soul mate, but you're f***ing nuts. You are the priority, I'll never leave you. If we don't have children, I can live with that, but if I don't have you … I can't live with that'. - **Brett**

This question is often asked of infertile people,

"So, whose fault is it anyway?"

It is a highly insensitive question and shows the ignorance of the person asking it. What they are clumsily trying to find out is, 'Do you have male factor or female factor infertility?'

Even then, the question doesn't cover all the possibilities. Infertility might be age-related, unexplained or social, as it is with homosexual parents-to-be.

And your diagnosis is none of their business.

Most importantly, don't blame yourself or your partner for your infertility. No one would deliberately choose to be infertile, so it is not your fault. If you do feel unresolved feelings of guilt or blame, forgive yourself. These emotions will not help you as you go on your infertility journey.

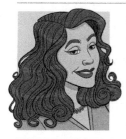

*Don't blame yourself for your infertility. 40% of the time it's male factor infertility, 40% of the time it is female factor and 20% of the time we may find something wrong with both of you, so in actual fact, it's 50/50. Be supportive of each other and don't blame yourself or each other. - **Dr Lynn Burmeister***

It is widely known that men can let a diagnosis of infertility affect their sense of masculinity. Some men will even let people think it is their partner who is infertile to avoid the stigma that they think will be associated to them. Many men are not able to talk about it, bottling up their emotions to perhaps cause issues down the track with unresolved grief and disappointment.

Once you have accepted the challenge of infertility as a couple, a single person or a baby-making team, the reason for your infertility becomes irrelevant apart from how it plays out medically. It is not helpful to anyone to focus on who is at 'fault'. Within a couple, assigning blame can only cause upset and resentment. Apologising and feeling guilty or getting angry and blaming will not help you conceive a child. It will only make you less resilient as a team. It can't be anybody's fault, because infertility is not something anyone can control.

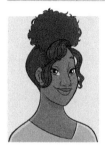

*When he got his azoospermia diagnosis, my partner kept constantly asking me if I was ok and apologising. I completely understand why he did this. It was a shock, he felt so guilty. I regularly reassured him it wasn't his 'fault' (and I meant it!) It's not like he did it deliberately! It meant that I felt I couldn't show my emotions or talk to him out of fear of upsetting him. He didn't want me to tell anyone else, so I internalised everything. I couldn't talk without him apologising to me. It built up so much anxiety and stress. I understand how he must have felt. It must feel awful feeling responsible, but the best thing he did was to accept that it wasn't his fault, it wasn't even in his control! We began to open up to family and friends and it gave me the space to process it myself. Once he stopped apologising, I could start to rely on him to be my support as we went through fertility treatment. - **Renee**

Assigning blame will not help you have a baby and it will not help you in your relationship. Make sure you use good language and terms like 'male/female factor infertility', although most of the time it is not even worth mentioning. Make sure you never allow anyone to describe your infertility as someone's 'fault' and make it clear to your partner that you shoulder this burden together, it is a shared diagnosis. When you decide to have a family with someone, your diagnosis becomes their diagnosis or vice versa. Once you decide to be a baby-making team, your diagnosis becomes your combined challenge.

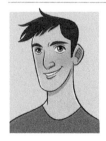

*We had a lot of hard times to start with because I was blaming myself for our infertility. But then my wife said to me, 'It's not your fault, don't be f***ing stupid!' Things got better when I realised it was a medical diagnosis and not my fault. - **Louis***

FROM LAURA

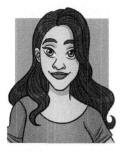 Jon has never apologised to me for his azoospermia. From the very beginning, he completely owned his diagnosis. He presented a 'take me or leave me' kind of attitude. If I chose to be with him, then infertility was part of the package. I must admit, it was initially kind of annoying, maybe I was hoping for some kind of dramatic apology for all I was going through with IVF.

Honestly, it was the best approach he could have taken. Neither of us could play the victim of his diagnosis and we could never use it to change the power dynamic within our relationship. He never felt guilty, and I never blamed him.

Occasionally, we would joke or make fun of each other. He would joke that I had signed up for this and I could trade him in for a man with good sperm and I would make fun of him and tell him to 'get some balls'. It lightened the mood that we could joke about it, knowing that there was never any blame associated with our diagnosis. It made me feel brave, I was choosing to take on infertility because I loved him so much. He never took me for granted because he was so grateful that we were facing this challenge together. It made us a much stronger team. And honestly, who could ever blame someone for having a medical condition?

BABY-MAKING MEET UP

After you receive a diagnosis (or if you are placed in the unexplained infertility category) connect in with your partner or your baby-making team.

▶ How are you each processing this new information? Allow your partner the opportunity to talk and feel the emotions surrounding what might be a significant shock.

▶ Remind yourself that infertility is just a puzzle to be solved. You may not know the answers yet, but you are on a journey of discovery and if you want to be a parent, you will find a way to be a parent.

▶ As you learn about your diagnosis, make sure your information comes from reputable sources. Don't go down an online searching rabbit hole! Together with your partner, work out a plan for researching your particular infertility diagnosis.

▶ Consider joining an online support group of people with the same diagnosis.

▶ Check in again with your Mindsets of Infertility – have you moved your position?

THE 7 MINDSETS OF INFERTILITY

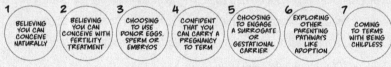

1	2	3	4	5	6	7
BELIEVING YOU CAN CONCEIVE NATURALLY	BELIEVING YOU CAN CONCEIVE WITH FERTILITY TREATMENT	CHOOSING TO USE DONOR EGGS, SPERM OR EMBRYOS	CONFIDENT THAT YOU CAN CARRY A PREGNANCY TO TERM	CHOOSING TO ENGAGE A SURROGATE OR GESTATIONAL CARRIER	EXPLORING OTHER PARENTING PATHWAYS LIKE ADOPTION	COMING TO TERMS WITH BEING CHILDLESS

Most of all, be kind to one another. You have been through a shock and it is important to allow yourselves space and time to process this new information.

See the Baby-Making Meet Up videos and download a workbook at www.InfertilityMan.com/MansGuide

LIFESTYLE CHOICES

When faced with a health challenge, most people would sooner look for a pill than make the necessary changes to their health and lifestyle. It takes a huge amount of dedication to change habits that have built up over a lifetime. It might seem easier to hand over all the power to a doctor with some magic medical protocol – until you figure out that they don't have a miracle cure either.

When you are handed a diagnosis of infertility, there are many areas of your life where you have the power to make a difference. Improving your eating and drinking habits, exercise routine (or lack thereof), recreational activities, lifestyle and mental health can all make an enormous difference. Infertility can make you feel out of control, but making improvements can give you back a sense of empowerment.

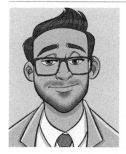

In IVF and conceiving, my belief is that every little bit helps. Who knows what that little extra 1% can do? When patients say to me 'Doctor, can I take supplements? Should I try to improve my diet? Can I do this or that?' I think it is worthwhile because there is some data to support these lifestyle changes in improving sperm parameters. You need the right environment for sperm to grow. Think of the cell that makes the sperm as a little seed and you want it to germinate, you want it to grow. You need the soil to be just right for that seed to sprout. The temperature needs to be right, everything needs to be in balance.

- Dr Darren Katz

When you are putting your money and energy into fertility treatment, you want to do all you can to ensure the best chance of success. Making lifestyle changes to improve your health and reduce your stress is a great way to look after yourself while undergoing treatment. The key is to make changes in a way that makes you feel good rather than deprived and restricted.

Your partner may be encouraging you to make lifestyle changes. Remember that she is only asking you to change because she is probably terrified. She's worried that you may never have a family, and that is a heavy thought. She may be making changes in her own life and it is frustrating for her to feel like it is not as important to you. Alternatively, she might not be making changes in her own life and asking you to lead the way because she doesn't know what to do.

Rather than seeing it as an annoyance, see it as an opportunity to show your caring and understanding. Infertility is a highly stressful experience, especially for women with a ticking biological clock. Be clear with your partner about which lifestyle changes you are willing to make and then follow through on your promise.

Improving your health and lifestyle is an ongoing process. There is little point in going to the gym once and expecting to lose weight. You have to keep going on a regular basis. When building new habits, you will have some days when you feel successful and some when you won't. Give yourself grace if you fall off the wagon. The worst outcome is to make a mistake and give up entirely. A better way is to notice that you have compromised your standards, dust yourself off and try again. Each time you will get better, if you just keep going.

Be kind to yourself and your partner, congratulate yourselves on any progress you make along the way and keep practicing until it becomes a habit. Practice doesn't make perfect; practice makes permanent. Anything you do repeatedly on an ongoing basis will eventually become a new habit, so make sure you are choosing the positive things to practice. Any progress is good progress.

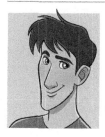

*It was a wake up call. My wife and I both changed our diets, and we dropped a lot of weight during IVF. She was having all those hormones pumped in, swelling and bloating. I don't know how she has managed, feeling like trash for four years. And now that we are pregnant, she's still feeling like trash. It doesn't stop. Makes you feel kind of lucky to be a man, but mostly it makes me want to look after her. The lifestyle and diet changes we made have stuck. We just value our health so much more after infertility. - **Liam**

THINGS TO AVOID

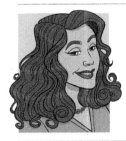

*We want Olympic athlete sperm; we want them to create Olympic athlete embryos that they will have the best possible chance of becoming a baby. If you are doing drugs, drinking alcohol excessively or making other poor lifestyle choices, you won't be creating Olympic athlete sperm. - **Dr Lynn Burmeister***

Stress

The most annoying thing you can ever say to someone trying to conceive is 'just relax, it will happen!' People struggling to get pregnant will not magically conceive just by relaxing. However, while relaxation will not automatically get you pregnant, being stressed out is certainly not going to help.

The body releases adrenaline when we're stressed, anxious or frightened. Unfortunately for many people, those are the emotions they experience when thinking about infertility. So what happens when you produce adrenaline? First, the heart rate will increase. Your body enters 'fight or flight' mode and will start pumping more blood to your arms (fight) and to your legs (flight), activating the sympathetic nervous system. When your body is in a constant state of physiological stress over perceived threats, its relaxation response doesn't always have time to kick in before the next stressor hits.

When trying to conceive it makes sense that your body needs to be in a receptive, relaxed and balanced state with the parasympathetic nervous system in control. It is best not to be in a state of fight or flight that many of us unconsciously live in. When we are relaxed, blood flow and energy is rerouted to the reproductive organs giving that system the resources it needs to function optimally.

Even if it is unclear whether stress is affecting your fertility, being too stressed may cause you to discontinue treatment. You may be so stressed out that you're not sleeping, eating properly, or exercising. If you need to take a break to manage your stress, that's ok. In the long run, taking care of your wellbeing and lowering your stress level is going to give you a better chance of successfully building your family, so do all you can to take care of yourself.

Alcohol

While research on how alcohol affects sperm has been mixed, we know that excessive drinking has a negative impact on health. An occasional drink may not have a major impact, but daily intake would certainly be a risk to your baby-making plans. It's not just about sperm either. Heavy drinking can affect your ability to get and maintain an erection, your sex drive and performance, which may make it harder for her to fall pregnant.

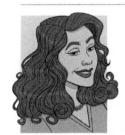

Excessive alcohol consumption has been shown to be detrimental to sperm health. If you can stop drinking altogether, that may be beneficial. Sperm takes three months to be created, so avoiding alcohol for that time before fertility treatment would be a good idea. Balance and enjoying your life is important, though any positive changes you can make may improve your chances of conceiving. - Dr Lynn Burmeister

For some people, it is easier to have a clear rule of no alcohol at all while trying to conceive, or at least in the three months before an IVF procedure. After you've had a few drinks, you're more likely to make poor decisions, not only with alcohol but with poor food choices too. Alcohol has no nutritional value and may derail any efforts you are making with your health. It is easier to cut back or stop drinking when the people around you are supportive, so you may choose to go alcohol-free to help your partner.

FROM JON

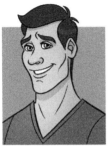

Our decision was based solely on the fact that drinking alcohol would not help us reach our goal of getting pregnant and having a family. We committed to remove alcohol from our lives while we were doing IVF. It was just easier for us to have a clear rule that we both followed. It was important to me to support Laura by not drinking, as I planned to continue to do if she got pregnant.

Smoking

You don't have to be a rocket scientist to know smoking does not lead to a healthy, happy, long life. So it stands to reason that it can have a negative effect on your fertility. Tobacco smoke contains harmful ingredients including nicotine, tar, carbon monoxide, polycyclic aromatic hydrocarbons and heavy metals. It reduces semen quality, decreases sperm count and causes erectile dysfunction. It elevates oxidative stress and DNA damage, which has a terrible impact on male fertility.

If you are honest with yourself, you already know that smoking harms you, your partner, your future children and all those around you. Hopefully, you plan to quit smoking in order to become a parent. No one wants to smoke around their kids. So why not start now? The desire to have a child could be the motivation that finally helps you to kick the habit.

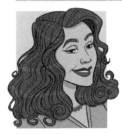

Smoking damages the DNA of sperm, which can create poor quality embryos. Even if your sperm looks ok during initial testing, smoking will still negatively affect the sperm's chance of creating quality embryos. Stop smoking if you are trying to have a baby.
- Dr Lynn Burmeister

Drugs

Illicit drugs have been proven to negatively affect your health and even occasional use can have a detrimental effect on your fertility. Not only can drugs cause erectile dysfunction, but they can also affect sperm shape and motility. There is research saying that it can affect the embryo and lead to miscarriage, premature birth and low birth weights.

Steroids and other performance enhancing drugs can cause the testicles to shrink and affect sperm production. Clearly, that is a disaster if you are trying to get your partner pregnant. It's a no-brainer, you shouldn't be using drugs while trying to conceive a baby.

Chemicals

Endocrine disrupting chemicals (EDCs) can reduce the quality of sperm and eggs and therefore affect the chance of becoming pregnant. The main EDCs are bisphenols (BPA/BPS/BPF), phthalates, parabens, heavy metals, pesticides, herbicides and insecticides. Most concerning is that there are around 800 artificial EDCs in everyday items such as plastics in food containers, personal care items, and food products. These chemicals can have negative effects on male and female reproductive health by mimicking or blocking hormones. Exposure to these chemicals can cause changes in hormone levels, decreased sperm and egg quality, damage to the DNA in sperm and cause an increased risk of miscarriage and early menopause.

The good news is that some simple changes can reduce your exposure almost immediately.
► Replace plastic food and drink containers with glass or aluminium.
► Wash your fruit and vegetables and buy organic when you can.
► Choose fresh, frozen or dried foods while limiting processed, canned and pre-packaged foods.

► Replace chemical laden household cleaning products with non-toxic alternatives.

► Replace personal care products that contain fragrances and parabens with non-toxic alternatives.

► Use stainless steel or cast iron cookware instead of non-stick.

Weight

Obesity in men can bring about hormone changes that affect sperm count. Excess weight has the potential to affect libido and cause erectile dysfunction. Many fertility clinics focus on the BMI in the female patient, but the male patient is equally important. There is a higher incidence of poor IVF outcomes when the male partner is overweight.

Even small amounts of weight loss, as little as a 10 percent reduction, can drastically improve your fertility outcomes. Taking control of this infertility puzzle piece has the added benefit of improving your quality of life at the same time.

Equally detrimental to your fertility goals is being underweight. Excessive exercise, stress and eating disorders can lead to infertility and adverse pregnancy outcomes. Women with a low percentage of body fat can experience challenges such as disrupted menstrual cycles and problems with ovulation.

Get Support

Making big changes in your life requires the right support. Reach out to get the help you need. Your GP can assist you, as can the many health professionals in the wellness industry. You may need to seek professional support to address the underlying psychological conditions that might be causing poor lifestyle choices. Your desire to have a family may be the motivation you need to move in a more positive direction.

FUEL YOUR BABY-MAKING MACHINE

Just imagine you are driving an expensive car, like a top of the range Ferrari. You have been hammering down the highway, top down, wind in your hair and the growl of the motor in your ears. You realise it is time to fuel up. You pull in and sidle up to the fuel pump, but instead of filling up with quality petrol, you walk into the service station and buy 60 litres of Coca Cola. You pour it in and fire that beast back up. Stupid, right? Why would you put Coca Cola in a Ferrari? If you want a machine to perform at its best, you need to give it the best fuel.

The same is true of your body. If you want it to perform optimally and produce the best possible sperm, give it the resources it needs.

Sacrificing junk food and Friday night drinks can be difficult, but at the end of your fertility journey you will want to know that you have given it your very best shot. One day, this period of your life will be over and if you want to go back to the bad habits then, you can. More likely, you will feel so good that you'll keep choosing your healthy lifestyle even after your fertility journey has ended.

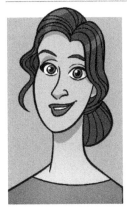

FROM TASHA JENNINGS
Fertility Naturopath and Nutritionist

Sperm is not just the DNA carrier we once thought it to be. Sperm health is involved in fertilisation, blastocyst formation, early embryonic development, miscarriage, pregnancy health as well as the lifelong health of your future child.

Having healthy levels of key nutrients and antioxidants through diet and appropriate supplementation can have a significant impact on your ability to conceive and carry your healthy baby.

There are several nutrients that can support sperm health. A Fertility Naturopath or Nutritionist can help make specific recommendations for you, however there are some that I find beneficial across the board.

Here's my top 5:

1. Zinc
Deficiency of zinc is associated with lowered testosterone levels, low sperm count and low sperm motility. Rectifying this deficiency through diet and supplementation has been shown to improve both these important factors and improve pregnancy outcomes.
Zinc is involved in the transformation of testosterone into its active form, which boosts available testosterone in the system.
It is best absorbed from animal sources as the phytic acid found in plant fibres can impair absorption. Vegetarians may benefit from supplementation. Supplementing with 20 – 40mg has been shown to be beneficial but do check your levels. A simple blood test can be ordered through your GP.

2. Coenzyme Q10 (CoQ10)

Co enzyme Q10 is found in significant amounts in seminal fluid. The amount of co enzyme Q10 present in seminal fluid has been found to be directly related to sperm count and motility.

CoQ10 is involved in the production of energy and is an antioxidant. Co Q10 is so vital to energy production and to life itself, our body naturally produces CoQ10 to support vital body functions. However, our ability to produce this natural coenzyme Q10 naturally declines as we age and demand for CoQ10 is increased by stress, illness and aging.

Therefore, getting enough through diet and supplements becomes more important as we age and during times of stress.

Supplementing 100 – 600mg can be beneficial. My general recommendation is 300mcg of the Ubiquinol form per day.

3. Vitamin C

Vitamin C is another antioxidant nutrient that is also found in seminal fluid helping to reduce oxidative stress and protect sperm from environmental damage. Good sources of vitamin C include oranges, kiwi fruit, grapefruit, blackcurrants,strawberries, cranberries, broccoli, cauliflower, sweet potato, tomatoes and loads more.

Supplementing 250 - 1000mcg per day can be beneficial. Vitamin C is water soluble and is lost from the body within 4 – 6 hours so I recommend divided doses over the day or 1 tsp in a bottle of water and drink over the day.

4. Lycopene

Tomatoes are also a wonderful source of lycopene, which is another antioxidant particularly important for male fertility.

Lycopene is one of the most potent antioxidants of all the carotenoids and is particularly useful for sperm health. The testes contain relatively high lycopene concentrations and low levels have been found in infertile men. It has been shown to reduce DNA damage and improve sperm count and viability.

Unlike most nutrients, lycopene is enhanced by cooking. So rich tomato pastes and sauces have more lycopene than fresh tomatoes.

Supplementation of 4 – 8mg for 3 months plus has been shown to improve sperm parameters and pregnancy rates.

5. Vitamin D

Vitamin D receptor enzymes and metabolising enzymes are found in the male reproductive system, particularly the testes. This important nutrient has been found to have a direct impact on spermatozoa and healthy levels are positively associated with sperm motility and fertilization.

Vitamin D levels should ideally be checked through your GP or specialist. Above 50 nmol/L is considered 'not deficient' however around 100 nmol/L would be a healthier level to aim for.

The best natural source of vitamin D comes from exposure to sunlight, however it's also important to be mindful of UV damage so supplementation is recommended if levels are low. Supplementing between 1000 – 5000IU per day can be beneficial depending on your levels.

To download Tasha's Fertile Pantry Checklist,
go to www.InfertilityMan.com/MansGuide

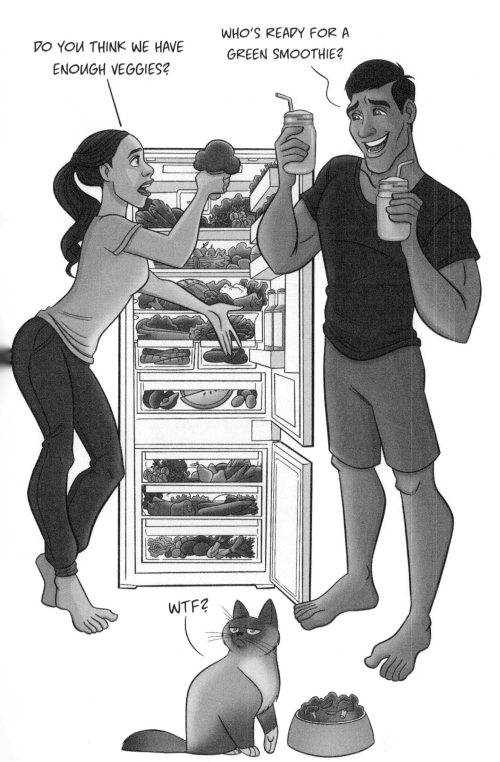

Diet

What you eat has a direct impact on how your body operates, especially on your hormones. A healthy diet has a positive impact on fertility and just makes you feel good.

'Decision fatigue' is the idea that when we have too many decisions to make, over time, our choices worsen. The psychological effects of decision fatigue can lead to difficulty making the good choices, impulse buying, impulse eating or other avoidance behaviours. The way to combat decision fatigue is to plan in advance, so you don't have to decide in the moment.

A good diet is all about being prepared. If you have already decided in advance what you are going to eat and drink, then you don't have to consider the unhealthy options.

A couple of tips:
► Maintain good hydration by always having a water bottle nearby to make sure you get the recommended amount.
► Replace sweets, lollies, cakes and biscuits with nuts, seeds, fruit & vegetables.
► Choose organic if possible.
► Replace processed foods by not having them in your house and instead buy fruit and vegetables.
► Replace your coffee intake with herbal teas.
► Make sure you have easy access to delicious natural food options, so you're not opting for fast foods.
► Find some great recipes that make you feel excited about healthy cooking.

It doesn't need to be complicated. Your chance to have children is a great motivation to make positive changes. While you may not be able to solve your fertility issues immediately, you can always improve your dietary habits and your lifestyle. It can be the one thing that you can control while living through all the uncertainty that infertility brings. Every change you make, even the small ones, can cause improvements in your fertility. Then you can rest easy knowing you have given it your best shot.

Exercise

There is ample evidence that exercise is good for our physical and mental wellbeing. The function of the reproductive system depends on the general health of the body, so when a man exercises regularly, the testicles may function better and sperm count may improve. If you are just starting out, any exercise is better than none. Walking, yoga and exercise classes can be a great way to begin.

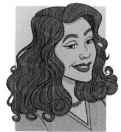

Sitting at your desk all day is not good for male fertility. As more men are living sedentary lifestyles, there does seem to be an increase in poor sperm test results. **- Dr Lynn Burmeister**

Exercise in a way that energises you rather than drains you. Your energy is needed to create sperm and high intensity or aggressive exercise can divert your energy away from your reproductive system. Exercise like intense cycling and triathlons should be practiced in moderation to avoid heating the testicles and causing physical stress on the body. More obvious forms of protecting fertility are important too, like wearing an athletic cup during high contact sport, avoiding saunas or upgrading to a better quality bicycle seat.

FROM JON

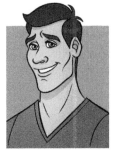

I don't like the word 'exercise', so I decided to change the words I used. Instead of gym and exercise, I began using words like movement, power, strength, flexibility and coordination as my buzz words to get me moving and motivated.

Besides these changes in my vocabulary, I don't make it wrong when I choose a particular type of movement over another. I don't make one type of exercise better than another, inevitably making me feel like I haven't achieved anything. This gives me every opportunity to win, rather than lose.

So on a busy day I might be headed to work and I don't have time for a full work out. Instead I do a short 15-minute routine at home, including strength, power, focus, coordination, flexibility and mindfulness. Even though I did not get to the gym that day I don't make it count any less in my mind. That box is ticked.

I guess it comes down to your ultimate outcome. Mine was to have a family with Laura. I knew I needed to maintain a healthy body to give any sperm I might have the best possible chance. It was great preparation for becoming a dad – feeling healthy, losing weight and being more mobile. I knew that one day, the little tackers were going to need me at my best.

Supplements

In addition to a healthy and balanced regimen of nutrition, supplements can help fill the gap or boost your levels of certain vitamins and minerals. It is best to create a supplement plan with healthcare professionals. Qualified nutritionists can perform blood tests and other assessments and create a plan to suit your situation and improve your fertility.

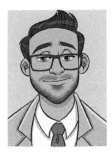

There is evidence that taking too many supplements can be harmful. I often see men coming in with a bag of supplements as they think 'more is better' – this is not correct. I favour the approach that a well-balanced multivitamin which is geared towards fertility is best. Only take as directed and don't take multiple different types. If anything else is to be ingested, it is important you speak to your complementary medicine practitioner and ask about the evidence for its use, as well as whether it interacts with any of the other supplements that you may be taking, bearing in mind that over-supplementation can be harmful even with 'natural substances'.
- Dr Darren Katz

FROM LAURA

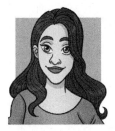

With the advice of a nutritionist and lots of research, I took a selection of well-chosen supplements in the lead up to my IVF cycles. My biggest tip: get a large pill box to sort your supplements and set alarms to remind you when to take them. On Sundays, Jon would get out the big box of bottles and fill up my pill box with all the vitamins and supplements I needed to take for the week. This was such a kind thing for him to do. If you are looking for ways to support your partner, this is a really great way to help.

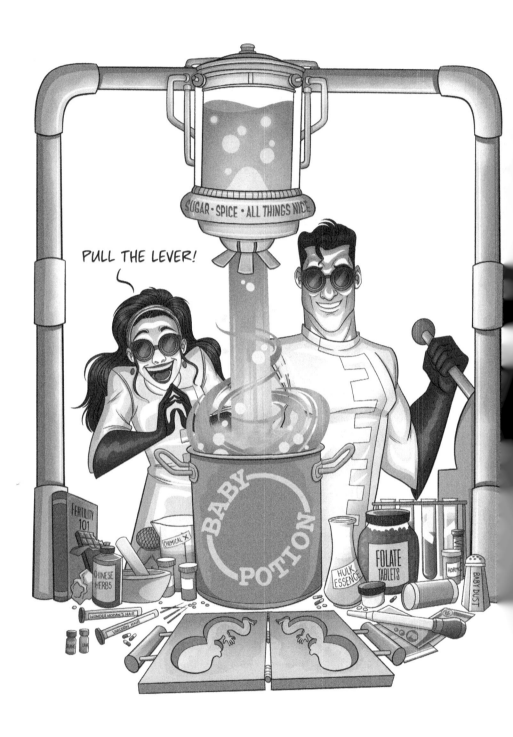

Sleep

Your circadian rhythm is your internally controlled timing device, which is affected heavily by your environment. Recent studies have found altered levels of FSH, LH, and prolactin may be caused by sleep disturbances or a disrupted circadian rhythm. Shift work, jet lag, and daylight savings time changes have been associated with poorer fertility and early pregnancy outcomes.

Restful, uninterrupted sleep is an essential part of your health routine. It is a challenge to get the required amount of sleep because there is so much distraction available to us now. Blue light from computer screens and digital devices can disrupt our circadian rhythm and lead to a poorer night's sleep.

A consistent sleeping routine and restful sleep environment provides the brain and body with the recovery time needed for optimum fertility.

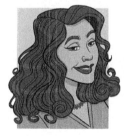

We know that lack of sleep causes poor egg and sperm quality. Melatonin is a great antioxidant and has been shown to be beneficial to fertility. **- Dr Lynn Burmeister**

Alternative Therapies

When it comes to infertility, it makes sense to use all the resources available to you. You may want to consider therapies such as chiropractic, acupuncture, osteopathy, Chinese medicine, massage, naturopathy, hyperbaric oxygen therapy or myotherapy.

While many holistic therapies aren't proven medically to aid fertility, many people report seeing great results. Whether it's the treatments themselves, the sense of being supported, or the feelings of wellbeing and calm that can result from these treatments, it is unknown which part does the patients so much good. What is known is this: if something seems to help you to improve your general wellbeing, it's a good idea to keep doing it!

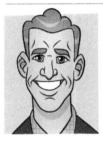

A subluxated spine/pelvis affects afferent and efferent nerve communications. Correcting these leads to a healthier spine and a healthy body.
- Dr Ryan Harrod, Chiropractor

KEEP YOUR BALLS COOL

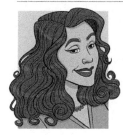 *I tell my guys to ice their testicles once a day. Get an ice pack, roll it in a towel and ice for twenty minutes a day while you're sitting, watching TV, just put it on your lap. It cools down the area and we know that overheating the testicles lowers the sperm count. Not too cold, don't get frostbite!* **- Dr Lynn Burmeister**

The testicles have two main functions: to produce sperm and to make testosterone. You may have heard that it is important to keep them cool. If they get too hot, it can affect the production and quality of sperm.

Approximately three degrees Celsius below normal body temperature is optimal for the production and storage of sperm. As you will know, your testicles will make a hasty trip inside when things get too cold and hang loose if they get too hot.

Avoid:
► Tight clothing and underwear
► Hot showers and baths
► Saunas
► Spa baths
► Sitting for long periods as contact with thighs generates heat
► Putting computers and other devices on your lap

Make a conscious effort to cool your balls:
► Wear boxer shorts instead of tight briefs
► Wear loose pants, jeans or shorts
► Have cool baths or showers
► Hop into the ocean for 10-15 minutes
► Apply ice to your groin (but do not put ice packs directly on your skin)

FROM JON

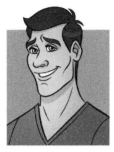

In the lead up to my surgeries, I made cooling my balls part of my daily routine. I wasn't a fan of a bag of peas (not comfortable and difficult to freeze again, though maybe you could make a soup afterwards). I preferred the soft gel ice packs because they would mould gently around my package, whereas the hard ones are, well, hard!

You can buy special ice pack underwear for exactly this purpose. After trying a few brands, I decided I preferred my own design. I would wear two pairs of shorts and put the soft ice pack in between. It worked perfectly and was comfortable enough to wear during my meditation in the morning and while watching a movie in the evening.

When it comes to lifestyle changes to enhance your fertility, you will need to have your own health assessed and do your own research. There are great fertility books written by doctors that go into more detail on topics such as diet and supplements. Create your plan and set alarms to remind you to execute on it. Use a pillbox to measure out your daily supplements – make it as easy as possible to take the correct amount every day. If you would like to see the lifestyle changes I implemented in the lead up to my sperm retrievals, go to www.InfertilityMan.com/MansGuide

We made changes to our lifestyle that made us feel like we were getting closer to our hopes of being parents. When we took away a particular behaviour, we aimed to replace it with a healthier behaviour so that we didn't feel deprived. These constant and never ending improvements have now become a way of life for us. Infertility will always be with us, because it caused us to make so many positive changes that will last for a lifetime.

BABY-MAKING MEET UP

Time for a catch up with your baby-making team. Emotions can run hot when discussing your health and lifestyle choices. It's important to focus on the changes that you want to make in your own life and not on forcing change on other people.

▶ What lifestyle changes do you each commit to in order to improve your fertility?

▶ Which people (friends and professionals) can help to improve your health?

▶ What resources (gyms, books, online programs) will you access to help to improve your health?

▶ Why is it important that you make these changes?

▶ What is your ultimate goal that will make it all worthwhile?

MENTAL HEALTH

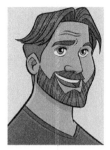

We did two IVF cycles back to back. The first one we started with sixteen early blastocysts, ended up with one, we transferred that but it didn't stick. Then we did a second IVF cycle straight away and we got eight or so eggs, and... zero made it. On Day 5, they told us 'nothing to freeze, nothing to transfer'. We were just absolutely ruined. It was so dark. **- Josh**

Infertility can have an enormous impact on emotional wellbeing. It can be a very frustrating experience and you never know how long you are going to be living with it, maybe months or even several years.

People faced with infertility report elevated levels of anxiety and depression, so it is clear that infertility causes stress. A comparative study (AD Domar, PC Zuttermeister and R Friedman) found that women who have problems getting pregnant experienced psychological symptoms similar to those associated with other serious medical conditions like cancer and heart disease.

Infertility can cause enormous grief over life not flowing as we expected it would. Not knowing how the future is going to be and whether you will be able to have children is hard. It can feel as if you are left out, watching other people experience the happiness of being parents. It can feel as if you are standing outside a window and only allowed to look in through it, but never enter.

Pregnancy loss and failed fertility treatments can bring about immense grief. Infertility can be pain, loss, questions, doctors, frustration, broken dreams, injections, heartache, waiting, weight gain, fear and disappointment.

Then there is hope. There is always hope, otherwise it would be impossible to keep going. Sometimes the hope can be the most confusing part of the whole experience.

Men are intensely impacted, though it may be difficult for them to share their feelings. Sometimes men feel they are not entitled to their negative emotions and they feel pressure to play a constantly supportive role to their partner.

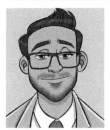

Males suffer, they really, really suffer through this. When a man is told he is infertile, it really hits him right where it hurts. Patients go through all the constellation of symptoms; depression, sense of loss, and it can affect their manhood. It's a real downer for lots and lots of men. It is such a roller coaster, so the support that you can get through the professional IVF services is just so important. I tell my patients that going and getting support from a counsellor is a sign of strength, not a sign of weakness.

Unfortunately, in my experience, there seems to be so much focus on the female when the male is deeply affected as well. So my shout out to all the people going through this is, don't forget the male in the picture, they're also suffering a lot of the time. - Dr Darren Katz

It is so important for men to acknowledge their own difficulties with infertility. How can you truly support someone else if you are not ok yourself? Make efforts to recognise and express your emotions, especially during the most challenging moments on your infertility journey. Not doing so can lead to ongoing mental health challenges.

When trying to conceive, you might also be concerned about the mental health of someone else, often your partner. Women share that infertility is one of the most challenging experiences of their lives. As well as experiencing difficult moments emotionally in their fertility journey, women may also have an adverse response to what is happening physiologically in their bodies. Fertility medications, intensified menstrual symptoms and changes due to pregnancy can all impact on a woman's mental health.

Note: Women with a history of sexual assault or women who have been through difficult experiences, such as having an abortion, may be particularly vulnerable during fertility treatment. Encourage her to seek professional support if she shows signs of disrupted mental health due to her past experiences.

The best way to support your partner is to proactively take care of your own mental health. Men often take a supportive role when a woman is struggling to conceive, but it is important to realise that this experience is happening to you too. Seeking appropriate support systems and building habits to take care of your emotional wellbeing is imperative as you navigate this difficult time.

Even though it may not be second nature to you, share how you are feeling. When men try to put on a brave face, women can misinterpret that and assume that they are disengaged. Women may see no acknowledgement of their pain and in turn, feel even more isolated and alone. It is so important to feel and show your emotions. You don't need to be strong all the time, it will most likely be better for your relationship if you allow yourself to be vulnerable.

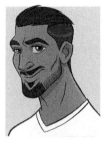

*I got to the stage where I just didn't want to think about it, because it bummed me out. I couldn't face it. It sounds strange, but I felt like I had lost somebody that I had never met. It seemed like we were giving up a dream that we had. We bought a new house and I was standing there in the empty rooms and I felt sad. We had a dream of filling all the rooms up. - **Justin***

If you are feeling depressed or anxious, there is help available. Reach out to your partner, family or friends – anyone who you feel might be able to lend an ear. Talk with your GP, they can refer you to a counsellor or psychologist. Realise that infertility is incredibly challenging and you will need to put measures in place to support your mental health. It takes a team to get through infertility and you must use all the resources available to you.

FROM JON

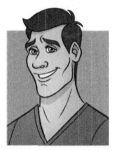 *Fertility stress can increase around certain days or events, especially for women who feel their biological clock ticking loudly. You or your partner may feel a bit down on your birthdays or Christmas or other holidays. You may feel conflicting emotions when people around you announce their pregnancies and it might be difficult to celebrate baby showers or children's birthdays. It might be a tough time when her period arrives each month. Anticipate these dates and be prepared to offer support to your partner and be extra gentle with yourself.*

Important: Sometimes it is appropriate to fall apart, cry, and feel the grief of infertility and pregnancy loss. We have more information about loss and grief later in this book.

And sometimes, it is appropriate to build resilience, focus on the positive, be optimistic and do whatever you can to move forward.

This chapter is focussed on building resilience, mindfulness and optimism, but it is not intended to minimise the very real pain that is part of an infertility journey. We want to give you some strategies to protect your mental health, but we are certainly not saying that it is simple when you have been through real trauma. If you are experiencing grief, loss or a particularly difficult time in your infertility experience, please read the chapter at the end of this book called 'Experiencing Loss'.

LIMBO

When you have apprehension about your reproductive future, it can put you and your partner into a state of limbo. Infertility can cause years of uncertainty. It might feel as if the appointments, planning, longing and dreaming are never-ending. You might find yourselves putting major decisions on hold, like starting a new job, moving house or taking an overseas holiday.

Some people even find small decisions challenging, like, should I eat this treat as it might affect my fertility? Or women might even think things like, why even bother trying to lose weight, as I might be pregnant again soon. Some may give up entirely and engage in self-destructive behaviour that doesn't help with their fertility goals.

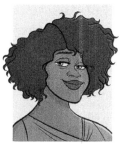

My husband and I found it valuable to resist the pull to live our entire lives in the waiting cycle that is infertility. We took vacations, we pursued new careers, we moved to another state. We didn't want to look back when it was all over, only to realise our lives were paused because of how badly we wanted to be parents. It's so hard to do, but look for ways that you can still love each other and build the lives you want together even while you're waiting for this next phase of your family.
*You will not regret it. - **Daria***

Acknowledge that you may be in this state of limbo for a while. Communicate with your partner so you can decide together whether decisions should be made with fertility in mind, or whether you should momentarily ignore your fertility issues and just make a decision that allows you to live your life more fully.

FROM LAURA

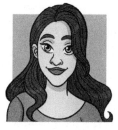

Fertility medications definitely affected my mental health while we were doing IVF. I think it is so important that partners understand just how much the drugs can alter a woman's mood and mental state.

Hormone medications can intensify premenstrual tension, causing symptoms like anxiety, confusion, depression and lowered mood, which may even include suicidal thoughts. Many women experience difficulties concentrating, memory lapses, a drop in self-esteem and confidence, a drop in sexual desire, or (occasionally) an increase, feelings of loneliness and paranoia, irritability, including angry outbursts, mood swings and weepiness. I look at that list and realise that I experienced all of them during our many IVF cycles.

During my first few cycles, I didn't really understand what was happening to me. I had several moments where I noticed I would react more than I would have if I wasn't taking hormone injections. As I became more experienced and did more IVF cycles, I noticed my emotions were closely tied to my menstrual cycle. I kept track of it, and perhaps the only benefit to doing seventeen IVF stimms cycles was that I started to notice patterns. Instead of just having random emotional outbursts, I could tell Jon in advance that I might be experiencing hormonal mood swings at certain times.

When both of us understood that this was happening, we could be more understanding of unusual emotional reactions and reduce some of the intensity. My advice, don't say to her 'you are clearly just hormonal!' That doesn't help her feel understood or supported. Don't push back, argue or disagree with her, even if she is completely in the wrong. Don't disconnect or leave. Be patient and trust that it will pass. Communicate to her that you understand her and that you love her. If you can, try to acknowledge that these are some pretty serious medications. Your kindness and empathy are honestly the most helpful thing to her in these moments. And of course, if you have concern for her safety or the safety of anyone else, please seek professional help.

PERSPECTIVE

There is an old story about two men who fought in the Vietnam War. They had a similar experience during the war, but the meaning they took from it was completely different.

On separate occasions, the two men watched as their best friends stood on landmines and were blown up. Both had horrific memories of this traumatic experience. However, there was one way in which these men differed from each other. They took a different meaning from this experience.

One man saw his best friend die in Vietnam and he took this meaning, 'Life is unfair. Man's cruelty to others knows no bounds. There is no beauty or joy in life, bad things happen to good people.'

The other man saw his best friend die in the same way and he took a different meaning. 'Life is short. People are willing to make the ultimate sacrifice to stand up for others. There is so much good in the world and I must live now to honour my friend.'

Same experience, different meaning.

Which of these two men do you think went on to be happier?

In a similar way, there are different ways to view fertility depending on the meaning you give it.

For example, 'This is so unfair. This problem is unsolvable. The odds are against us, I'll never become a parent. Other people get pregnant so easily, it's not fair. There must be something wrong with me. Why even bother trying?'

Alternatively, fertility challenges may be viewed like this, 'This is a challenge but we can figure it out together. We have access to incredible medical support and we will find a solution to this puzzle. Facing this challenge together will bring me closer to my partner and make us stronger. And one day, we will be better parents because of this experience. We may not be able to conceive a child naturally, but we can find a way to become parents if we want to be. Over time, we could also choose to remain childless and still have happy and fulfilling lives. I'm ready for this.'

THE ARGUMENT FOR OPTIMISM

Infertility is a tough experience to live through and it can certainly have a negative impact on the mental health of you and everyone in your baby-making team.

However, there is a difference between feeling the emotional pain of infertility and living in constant suffering. Having a focus on the negative will not make you strong enough to meet the gruelling experience of infertility and IVF treatment. Our brains, when undirected, will always tend to focus on the hassles, the stresses, the complaints and the difficulties that infertility presents in our lives.

Of course, there will be moments in your fertility journey when it will be appropriate to feel sad. Feeling emotions fully helps us to process negative experiences and is vital for good mental health. The question is, will being sad for a long period of time change anything? If the answer is no, then you should have a think about how much time you should devote to feeling sad. Reach out for support to process your emotions, so that you can get back to moving forward.

We may believe that if we are successful at conceiving a baby, then we'll finally be happy. Our brains work in the opposite order. If we can find ways to be happy while going through infertility, the optimism we feel will make us more resilient and better equipped to face the challenges of fertility treatment.

If you can raise your level of positivity in the present, then your brain will experience what can be called a happiness advantage. Your brain in a positive state performs significantly better than it does in negative, stressed or neutral. Your intelligence, your creativity and your energy levels rise.

With increased optimism, you will have an increased ability to see stress as a challenge instead of a threat. Infertility is usually a long-term challenge and a positive attitude can only help you as you progress through it.

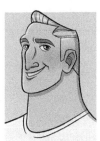

My wife and I are on IVF round 7. What an emotional rollercoaster!! Far out! Enough to do your head in sometimes. You need resilience to get through this crazy, testing, unbelievably hard - but do-able with a strong mindset – ride. **- Anthony**

SELF-CARE

Be proactive in taking care of your own mental health. Use exercise to clear your head. Read books that help you remain calm and focused. Talk to people who make you feel good. Consciously think about things you're grateful for. Laugh as much as you can. Meditate, eat healthily and sleep. Breathe. You know what to do to take care of yourself. Many of these activities are available to you at any time of the day, wherever you are. Make a conscious effort to bring healthy habits into your everyday life.

Right now, you need to be like an athlete, because this is a marathon. Athletes have routines and thought processes to keep them in a focused mental state. You need to take care of yourself like you were preparing for the most important race of your life... because you are.

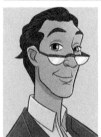

*We're pregnant now. It wasn't as long a road for us as for some. We're very thankful for that. It still felt like 100 years though. - **Matthew***

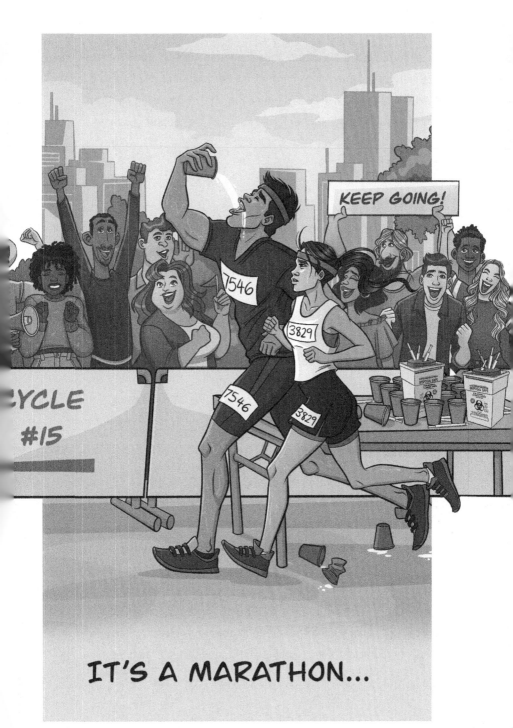

IT'S A MARATHON...

Counselling

Many fertility clinics provide counselling. Sometimes it is even a requirement that you go to counselling in order to begin treatment. If counselling is available to you, use it! Even if your clinic doesn't provide it, seek out a counsellor who specialises in fertility and get the support you need.

Support Groups

Join a fertility support group, either online or in your community. Pay attention to whether these groups make you feel good as sometimes people come together to just share in more misery. The majority of these groups have a very positive focus and can provide advice and support that only comes from having lived through similar experiences.

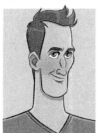

*You don't start talking about it until you are in it and then you realise how little it is spoken about. But you come to realise how much you are not alone and your journey is not so unique. Infertility is so much more common than you realise when you start out. - **Sam***

Meditation

By turning your attention away from distracting thoughts and focusing on the present moment, meditation has been shown to reduce stress. As well as making you feel good, meditation may have a positive impact on fertility.

There are so many guided meditations, apps and videos available to begin a meditation practice. Keep it simple and start with just 10 minutes a day.

FROM JON

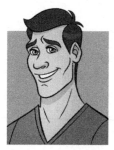

The morning and the night are my time for mindfulness. The morning is for gratitude and preparing for the day ahead, and the evening is for reflection and letting go. I remember starting my meditation practice years ago, and I could only focus for a minute at a time. I honestly couldn't sit for any longer than that. As time went on, I have pushed it out to 10 minutes in the morning and 10 minutes in the evening. I started to look forward to my meditations each day and enjoy it.

My routine will be forever known as my 'bits'. Laura gave it this name when she realised how important it was to me.

"Hey Jon, are you doing your bits now?"

She would realise if I didn't answer, it was because I was doing my meditation. She always gives me space during my meditation time because she knows it makes me even more present when she needs me to be.

As we made our way through fertility treatment, I would focus on what I hoped to achieve. I would think about what I wanted, namely sperm. Lots of sperm. And not just any sperm, buff little bad boys in training, and training hard. I would imagine them doing push-ups, shoulder stand press ups, bench press and crunches. I decided that if my doctor was going to find sperm then they would be the in the best possible shape. I would imagine them in my mind, swimming in races. I found that the more entertaining my meditations, the more composed I was for our tougher days. Who knows whether it helped us to find the sperm, I like to think that it did!

Try out a Meditation for Male Fertility at www.InfertilityMan.com/MansGuide

Breathing

Just breathe… easier said than done sometimes, especially when trying to conceive. Breathing can be used to centre you and help to regain that control when you're feeling overwhelmed. The best part about it, you can do it anywhere, anytime, anyplace and it's completely free. Since you have to do it anyway, might as well breathe deeply and use it as a tool to make you feel good.

FROM JON

I sit and make myself comfortable (sitting on a pillow helps), close my eyes (optional), and focus on my breath, in and out through my nose. The reason I keep my mouth closed is that I feel nasal breathing slows me down even more.

There are lots of different breathing techniques that can help to ease stress. Triangle Breathing consists of imagining each breath cycle as a triangle, using a 4:4:4 ratio for inhaling, holding, and exhaling.

Breathe in (count to 4)
Hold (count to 4)
Breathe out (count to 4)

With practice, you can increase to a 4:8:8 ratio.

Breathe in (count to 4)
Hold (count to 8)
Breathe out (count to 8)

This is my favourite relaxation technique and you can do it anywhere, especially when you need to quiet the chatter in your mind and come back to the present moment.

RESILIENCE

In his article "Three Steps to Resilience", Hugh van Cuylenburg describes how his trip to India taught him a lesson in resilience. He wrote that it seemed that the people he met there, despite their more difficult living conditions, seemed to have found the secret to happiness and resilience.

He says, ultimately, there were three principles the villagers in India practiced every day that were key to their resilient world view and cheerful disposition:

▶ Gratitude (the ability to pay attention to what you have instead of worrying about what you don't have)
▶ Empathy (the ability to feel what another person is feeling)
▶ Mindfulness (the ability to focus on the present moment).

The villagers faced daily hardships and pressures, often more acute than most of ours in the west, but they managed their responses differently.

These concepts can be applied to fertility and shared with your partner if they are struggling. You are gearing up for a challenging journey, so this is a time in your lives when you may have to be even more proactive in making sure you keep your resilience. You will have to do certain things, pay attention to certain things (and ignore others) and think consciously in order to navigate the stresses ahead. Be proactive in strengthening your mental health.

THE IDEAL INFERTILE PEOPLE

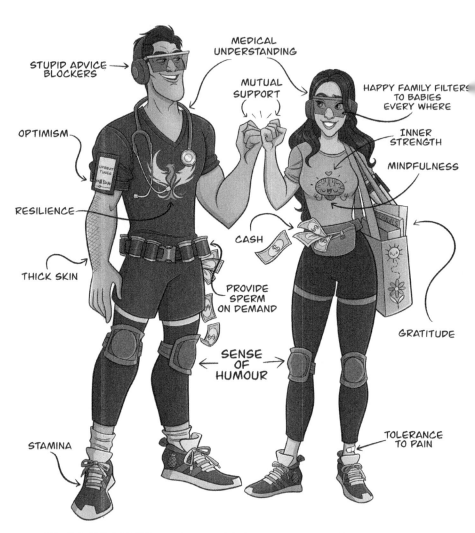

PLEASE NOTE: IDEAL FERTILE PEOPLE CAN BE ANY GENDER, SINGLE OR IN ANY KIND OF RELATIONSHIP.

To have the stamina to keep going through the challenges of infertility, you will need to actively build your resilience. Negative thinking and unkind feelings towards others and yourself will only weaken your resolve and make it even more difficult for you to stand up to the rigours of fertility treatment.

Make conscious efforts to build your resilience.

1. Gratitude. Write in a journal every morning or night, listing three things that you are grateful for that day, even if they are very small. Focusing on what you have, rather than what you don't, will help you feel even more peaceful. This simple activity will allow you to relive the positive aspects of your day and train your brain to scan, not for the negative, but for the positive.
2. Empathy. When you feel down, do a small act of kindness. Send a friendly message or a gift and pay someone a compliment. It will make you feel good. Give with no thought of receiving something back in return.
3. Mindfulness. Practice being present in whatever task you are doing, even housework like folding clothes or washing dishes. Take up a hobby that requires your full attention. Meditate. Actively put activities into your life that help you be in the present moment.

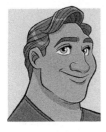

Our mindset during infertility went like this:
Naïve, hopeful, shocked, confused, developed a plan,
seemed like it would take forever, coming closer to the
end, but still like it would take forever, more certain
and confident, then hopeful again. You will get there.
*Just keep moving forward. - **Leo***

BABY-MAKING MEET UP

It's time to have a very important conversation with your baby-making team. Taking care of your mental health is paramount as you navigate infertility. You must actively work to improve your positivity and emotional wellness, otherwise infertility will certainly bring you down.

Resilience and self-care will give you the stamina to keep going as you work hard to build your family. You deserve to be happy in the meantime, so you must be proactive in looking after your partner and yourself.

Limbo

► Is there an area of your life that you have been putting on hold while you have been struggling with infertility?
► How can you step out of infertility limbo and live your life right now?

Perspective

Dig deep and find the positive meaning for your infertility. Write it down. Imagine yourself in the future when you have solved this puzzle.
► Who have you become?
► How have you grown?
► How are you better as a person because of what you have been through?
► What good can come from what you are experiencing right now?
► Who will you be able to help in the future because of what you are learning now?
► What are you grateful for in your life right now?

This is so challenging to do, but one day in the future you will look back on your fertility journey and see positives, so why not start now?

Self-Care

▶ In your life, are there areas where you could take better care of yourself?

▶ Which hobbies or activities make you feel good?

Create a Menu of Ways to Feel Good. Make sure you have options on there that you can do any time, any place and that don't require a lot of planning, money or other people. Make it easy to feel good.

PREPARING FOR TREATMENT

In most cases, one person on your baby-making team will do loads of research and preparation. They will read lots of fertility books, sign up for all the websites and message boards, and by the time you get your diagnosis, they are ready. By contrast, the other partner just seems to fumble along, not really sure what the procedures are, what they are supposed to do or even any intelligent questions to ask.

The fact that you are reading this book makes you more switched on and more engaged than the average guy. You are preparing to face this battle head on. You are preparing like all good warriors, because you know that your mental state is what wins the war.

History has shown that the greatest battles make the greatest heroes. You truly grow into the best that you can be when you face adversity head on. You are about to become a Fertility Superhero. If you are to be the Fertility Superhero that your baby-making team needs, then you need to prepare for this important role.

Stephen Covey wrote a book called *The Seven Habits of Highly Effective People*, which sold over 25 million copies. Along with brilliant habits such as Be Proactive, Begin with the End in Mind and Seek First to Understand, he described Habit Number 7: Sharpen the Saw.

The idea goes like this: A woodsman was asked, "What would you do if you had just five minutes to chop down a tree?" He answered, "I would spend the first two and a half minutes sharpening my saw."

People sometimes get swept up in an 'infertility journey' and it feels like they are suddenly on a rollercoaster that is speeding out of control.

Preparation is key and you are going to take a few specific steps now (even if your journey has already begun) to be as prepared as you can be. This is especially important if your partner is significantly impacted by this experience emotionally. By stepping up, engaging and preparing for what lies ahead, you are creating a solid foundation for yourselves that will give you the best chance of managing the stressful experience ahead.

This chapter includes some simple steps that you can act on immediately. Once you realise you are headed into fertility treatment, it is so important that you are prepared and on the same page with your partner.

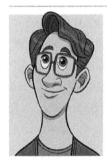 *We decided to keep trying naturally while making lifestyle changes, but if we weren't successful by the end of the year, we would move to IVF. We initially thought that IVF wasn't for us, but it is funny how the things you thought you wouldn't do, you find yourself doing real quick when you start to want something that you didn't really know that you wanted so badly. - Ian*

RESEARCH

Having any serious medical diagnosis is a steep learning curve. Infertility is particularly tricky to navigate because each person's diagnosis can be vastly different. Even if you have friends who have struggled to conceive, how they were treated medically is probably quite different from what you are experiencing.

FROM JON

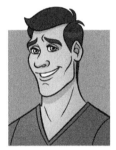

Laura is definitely more of a nerd than me, so she really got into researching about infertility. She would talk to me about the things she was learning, which was easy because all I had to do was listen to get all the useful info I needed. It was also up to her to do most of our IVF treatment, which was a huge task in itself.

So, it became my job to work additional shifts at my job as a paramedic to bring in the extra cash we needed to pay for the medical appointments. At home, I would do extra cleaning and household chores when she was unwell during treatment. My biggest job was providing emotional support and a listening ear during the process.

We were a good team.

When you're experiencing infertility, you can absolutely expect help from doctors, nurses, friends and family. However, you must participate in your own rescue. You can't just hand over all responsibility to your doctor and hope for the best. No one else is ever going to care about your future family as much as you do, so you are the best person to direct your fertility treatment and make the big decisions. You must participate in your own rescue and to do that, you must be informed.

Think of it like this: Pretend you have fallen out of a boat in a rough ocean and you're drowning. The people on board are throwing out life jackets and floating rings to you. What must you do? You need to swim towards the life-saving devices, grab on and try to get yourself back on the boat. If you just stay still and wait for someone else to rescue you, you will surely drown.

There are many informative books, websites, support groups and people online who can help you learn about your infertility diagnosis and to understand and manage it. There are also some resources that can misinform you. Sometimes your research can make you feel empowered and prepared, and sometimes it can make you stressed and overwhelmed. You and your partner should come up with a plan for where and how you will get your information. Make conscious choices about which people and ideas you allow to influence you as you move forward in your infertility journey.

PAPERWORK

There is a lot of paperwork that goes along with fertility treatment. As you fill in all the forms, you will be asked some pretty intense questions about topics you have never considered before.

► Who are you granting access to use your eggs or sperm and under what circumstances?
► What will happen to any frozen eggs, sperm or embryos if you or your partner die?
► What will happen to any frozen eggs, sperm or embryos if you and your partner separate?

Although you don't have to decide this yet, the paperwork may cause you to think about what might happen to any leftover embryos at the end of your treatment. At this stage, you should just freeze them, but in the future you may give them to another family, donate them to science or discard them.

You will sign consent forms that describe the potential side effects, risks and potential consequences of fertility treatment. These include symptoms such as bloating, bruising, nausea, fatigue, headache, breast tenderness, upset stomach, hot flushes, mood swings and allergic reactions. You also sign up to potential consequences like pelvic infections and ovarian hyperstimulation syndrome (OHSS). You will acknowledge the increased risk of ectopic pregnancy and multiple pregnancy (twins, triplets or more). Consent forms will need to be signed for each cycle and each subsequent cycle.

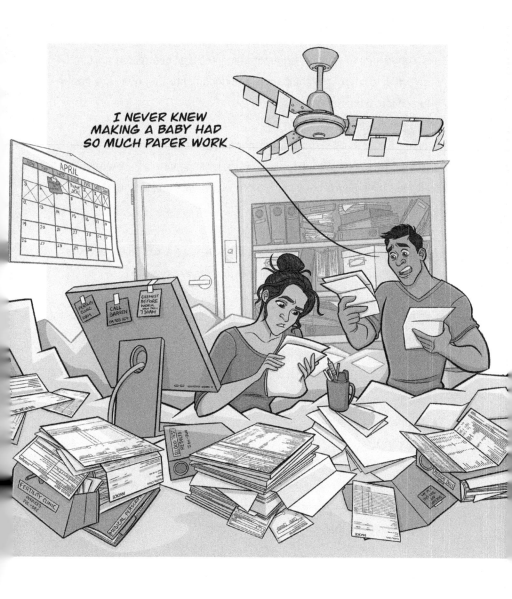

Fertility Folder

It is a good idea to have a system for managing it all before you start, rather than trying to sort out all the papers and documents after you have gotten yourself into a mess.

Create a folder, both on your computer and an actual binder with plastic pockets. You need somewhere that you can file paperwork – it works well if it is portable, as you may want to take it with you to your doctor's appointments.

This is such a simple thing to set up and it will make a lot of difference to your baby-making team to have all the paperwork organised.

Get a large binder and fill it with plastic pockets and dividers. Create several sections inside the folder with these titles:
► Blood Tests
► Finances
► Medications
► Supplements
► Insurance
► Cycles

Replicate the same system in your computer files. You may need more as you go along, but that is a great place to start.

Once this system is set up, it makes it easy for you to keep everything together. Even when you are on the go, if you get some papers from the doctor, an invoice in the mail or just pick up a pamphlet that you think will be useful, throw it in the folder. Make sure you write 'PAID' on any invoices you have already taken care of.

FROM JON

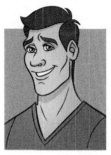

When we started IVF, we (naively) thought that we would be done and pregnant in one month. This was very much not the case. As it stretched out into several years, we were really glad that we had this system in place to keep all the papers organised. It was handy when we needed to look back at our history, for example comparing blood test results and telling doctors about medications we had used in previous cycles.

Fertility Summary

Believe it or not, one day you may not remember everything that happened on your fertility journey. Hopefully, your fertility treatment will be quick and successful, but more often than not, it takes some time and quite a few steps to get to your long-awaited pregnancy. It will be helpful if you can remember your own history; the details of your IVF cycles, your medications, your fertilisation results, and all the little steps along the way. It is helpful if you can recall them easily when speaking with doctors and other medical professionals.

So, it could be useful to create a document to track the key details of your fertility treatment. You would do it on your computer or on the top page of your fertility paperwork folder.

Example Fertility Summary

- ► December 2022: IVF Cycle #1, cancelled due to 6 follicles, Menopur 337.5 and Orgalutran 250
- ► February 2023: Natural pregnancy, miscarriage #1 at 5-6 weeks
- ► July 2023: IVF Cycle #2, Puregon 300, Menopur 140, Orgalutran 250, 7 eggs retrieved, 3 blastocysts frozen

Download a Fertility Summary printout at www.InfertilityMan.com/MansGuide

Fertility Calendar

When you first start fertility treatment, you think it will be a predictable timeline from where you are now (infertile) to where you want to be (pregnant). You plan out your dates, thinking that you will be pregnant by this date and have a baby by that date. A lot of the time, it doesn't happen that way you planned.

You will need a way to keep track of your dates, such as doctor's appointments and estimated IVF cycle dates. Most of this will have to be set up by the woman, as it will coincide with her menstrual cycle, but it is important that you stay linked into which dates you need to be available.

A shared online calendar or a simple wall calendar works beautifully for this. You can have a little code, where she can indicate which appointments she needs you to be there for and which appointments she is happy to handle by herself (keeping in mind that this may shift and change depending on how successful your treatment is and how you are both tracking emotionally).

FROM JON

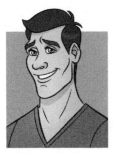

Our fertility treatment kept extending. It got to the point that it was futile to predict or even guess anything, not when we'd be pregnant, not when we'd start injections, not when we would have an egg pick up, not even when a period would start. We thought at the start that we would do one round of IVF and that would be enough. We ended up doing fifteen! It became difficult to plan trips, book flights, accept invitations and even hold down a job!

We found that a shared wall planner helped us to keep track of what might happen, and we were both constantly updating it. At least then we had some kind of idea when her periods were going to start, when she might begin injections, when we might be having surgery. It changed all the time, but at least we had a rough idea that we shared between the two of us.

PREPARING FINANCIALLY

Fertility treatment is a huge financial commitment. It can be very expensive and there is no guarantee that it will work. No doubt you already realise this and perhaps you are freaking out a little about it.

Think of it this way, would you ever hand over thousands of dollars to a mechanic who wasn't sure he could fix your car? What if he said that he had a 40 percent chance of fixing your car?

Fertility treatment is a big gamble, but the potential prize is worth the risk. The best you can do is take the most calculated risks and save money wherever possible. Comparing prices, finding value for money, choosing the best doctors, actively participating in your treatment and doing everything you can to take care of your health will give you the best chance of ensuring that your fertility money is well spent.

Fertility doctors and their teams should be paid well. Their jobs are demanding, and they are literally performing miracles every day. On the other hand, it is important for you to realise that you are paying them very good money and you have the right to expect excellent support.

The interesting thing about fertility treatment is that paying more doesn't necessarily give you more chance of bringing home a baby. Sometimes the better doctors are cheaper and sometimes they're more expensive. Often the really good doctors have reasonable prices but extremely long waiting lists.

You will need to get informed, do your research, and make smart decisions. Depending on your particular fertility issue, you may be able to choose a cheaper clinic, but still get a great result.

Saving and Budgeting

In most countries, fertility treatment costs money. You will need to have a plan in place for how you are going to come up with the cash to pay the doctor's bills, plus any incidental costs along the way.

For many couples, this can be an incredibly difficult part of their infertility experience. When you are already going through a challenging time emotionally and physically, financial stress can add a huge amount of additional pressure.

Everyone will be in a unique situation, so here are some questions to ask yourself.

► What can you do to prepare financially for your fertility journey?
► What changes can you make to your income or your expenses to keep yourself afloat financially as you pay for your treatment?

We almost always find ways to pay for things that we deem to be really important. If you become a parent, you won't regret the money that you spent to get there. However, it doesn't always work out how you want, so it's useful to really think about how much money you are willing to commit, remembering that your treatment plan and chance of success may change over time. No one else can decide this for you.

Healthcare and Government Support

Every country in the world has a different healthcare system and you may have government financial support for assisted reproductive technology (ART). You will need to do your own research into what is available to you in your location. Your fertility clinic will be able to provide some insight and you should also search for information online. Be aware that you might be eligible for different levels of support, depending on your diagnosis.

Insurance

If you have private health insurance, check what they cover when it comes to fertility treatment. Contact them and get clear information about what is covered in your policy. If you don't have private health insurance, do your research as you may determine that it works out better financially to start a health insurance policy once you factor in fertility costs. Do the research to ensure that you are adequately insured.

In some places in the world, working in a fertility friendly company is a good way to get insurance. Many people intentionally choose to work at these companies in order to have adequate coverage for IVF and other fertility treatments.

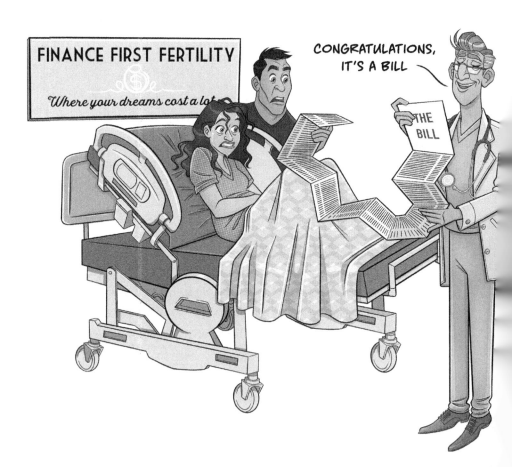

Important: Many health insurance funds have waiting periods for assisted reproductive technology and pregnancy. Even if you are not quite ready to start fertility treatment, add this extra to your policy as soon as possible so you have time to serve the waiting period. With any luck, you'll be ready to use it for a pregnancy if fertility treatment becomes unnecessary.

Budget

The clinic should provide written information about the costs of your treatment. If they don't, request it before you start treatment. Depending on the way your clinic is set up, you might receive separate invoices from your hospital, anaesthetist or embryologist, so make sure you include them in your budget. Some things are considered additional treatments, so don't be surprised if they are on a separate invoice. Ask lots of questions so you don't get any unexpected surprises.

Think about anything else that you or your partner may choose to spend money on to support your fertility treatment, such as acupuncture or supplements. Create a budget to make sure you agree about how you will spend your money. Below are some ideas of expenses you may need to include in your budget.

Fertility Costs

► Initial and follow up consultations
► Preliminary fertility testing and semen analysis
► Fertility medications
► Intrauterine Insemination (IUI) and other lower tech treatments
► Ultrasound monitoring and blood work during your cycle
► Testicular sperm extraction
► IVF egg retrieval and transfer
► Hospital costs

► Anaesthetist costs
► Intracytoplasmic Sperm Injection (ICSI) or Intracytoplasmic Morphologically Selected Sperm Injection (IMSI) (see Glossary)
► Assisted hatching
► Embryo testing
► Semen, egg and embryo freezing and storage

Additional Expenses

► Transport
► Accommodation
► Supplements
► Acupuncture
► Chinese Medicine
► Massage
► Ice packs
► Counselling
► Nutritionist
► Gym Membership
► Books or online courses

Download a Fertility Budget Template at www.InfertilityMan.com/MansGuide

PREPARING PHYSICALLY AND EMOTIONALLY

It is recommended that lifestyle changes be put in place at least three months before you start your fertility treatment. Considering how much money and effort you will put into your treatment and how much you want to conceive a child, it makes sense to give yourself the best possible chance. So ask yourself, what lifestyle changes do you need to put in place right now to prepare your body?

You will most likely know immediately what needs to change, it's not complicated, if you are really honest with yourself. You might need to quit smoking, eat less sugar, or take a break from drinking coffee. When you have an important reason like conceiving a child, it can feel really good to make positive changes for your health. Do the things that make you feel empowered, rather than stressed or deprived.

Hopefully, things will go perfectly and you'll have a baby on the way in no time. Unfortunately, fertility treatment rarely works right away. It can take time to get the correct diagnosis and then to get the treatment plan right. Even when everything looks perfect, it can still take several attempts before it works. Realistically, it might not go well for you initially. And there is certainly a chance that you may not conceive a baby at all, in which case you might choose to consider other ways of becoming a parent. Hope for the best but prepare for the worst.

It is so important for you and your partner to be resilient and emotionally prepared. Have a plan for when things don't go well. What people, places, things and activities can help you when this journey gets difficult? Create a list of resources that will help you along the way.

MENU OF WAYS TO FEEL GOOD

PEOPLE	PLACES	THINGS	ACTIVITIES
· Counsellor	· Ocean (to clear my head)	· Blender (for healthy smoothies)	· Going for a run
· Nutritionist	· Gym	· Journal	· Listening to music
· Sister	· The park near our house	· Weights at home	· Meditating
· Acupuncturist			
· Manager at work			

BABY-MAKING MEET UP

With your baby-making team, discuss the steps you need to take
to prepare for what lies ahead of you.

Research

▶ Which books, websites and online resources could help you understand
more about fertility treatment?

▶ Which of you will take the time to gather and understand the
information?

▶ How will you share the information?

▶ What is the best use of your preparation time?

Paperwork

▶ Create a system for your fertility paperwork, a physical folder to store
papers and a shared digital folder for storing online documents.

▶ Create a fertility calendar. Decide how you will share information about
important dates and appointments.

Finances

▶ What changes do you need to make to ensure you can pay for your
fertility treatment?

▶ Who will manage the financial aspects of your fertility treatment?

▶ Find out about any government rebates or assistance.

▶ Contact your private health insurance fund. Make sure that you have
Pregnancy and Assisted Reproductive Technology included in your policy.
Find out about any waiting periods and mark those dates on your
fertility calendar.

▶ Create a fertility budget to forecast your expected costs.

▶ Compare costs for different clinics and doctors and ensure that you
are happy with your choice.

Physical and Emotional

- ► Do you need to make changes to your lifestyle?
- ► What do you each commit to improving right now?
- ► How will you cope if things don't go as you expect?
- ► How do you prefer to be supported in difficult times? How can you rely on each other?
- ► What resources will you draw on in tough times? For example, counselling or therapy, journaling, support groups.

PREPARING YOUR SUPPORT CREW

In addition to your baby-making team, you will need an entire group of people to support you. Your Support Crew might include medical professionals like doctors and nurses; complementary therapists like nutritionists and acupuncturists, as well as family, friends and other people who have already been through fertility treatment. These people will work for you and with you to give you the information, medicine and tools you need to complete your mission. They may also provide the emotional support you will need along the way.

► Who are the people in your Baby-Making Team?
► Who are the professional and personal contacts that will be in your Support Crew?

Choose compassionate people in your life, tell them what you are going through, and ask for their support.

Important: You need to have a conversation with your baby-making team about your privacy as you go through fertility treatment. If you tell everyone, the questions and comments might be overwhelming, whereas, if you tell no one, you might feel isolated and alone. Confirm with your team how private they would like to be; perhaps they want to tell no one, or just some family and friends. Some people are very private. Others are very open and share lots of details about what they're going through.

It might be helpful to have certain people in your workplace know you are seeking fertility treatment. You may need to take time off work to go to the doctor or you may have periods of being unwell or recovering from surgery. Or it might be best to keep it private from your employer.

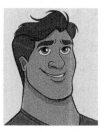

*My work colleagues were ridiculously supportive. They went over and above, giving me flexibility, support, whatever I needed. It meant I could go to every doctor's appointment. I was there every time my wife had surgery and the days afterwards for her recovery. If she was having a day or a week where she was struggling mentally and I didn't want her to have to be on her own, I just worked from home and none of it was an issue. - **Will***

Some people are comfortable sharing what they are experiencing on social media, whereas that would mortify others. It is so important that you, your partner and anyone else involved are comfortable with the level of privacy. Respect the boundaries of everyone involved in your fertility journey.

FROM JON

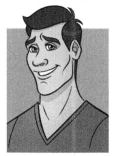

Initially, we didn't tell anyone that we were starting IVF. We went through our first year without sharing with anyone at all. I think we had this romantic idea that it would work quickly and then we could just announce that we were pregnant and no one would know how the baby was conceived.

As our fertility treatment went on (and on), we wanted more people to know what we were going through, even if they didn't really understand. In our second year, we talked about the best way to share our infertility experience. We realised we needed some support. It was becoming too challenging to keep the secret and we needed to reach out for help. We had some one-on-one conversations with family and friends. Soon we had a small group of people we felt comfortable confiding in.

Sometimes these conversations went well but sometimes, we walked away feeling worse. Suddenly we felt overwhelmed by having to explain how IVF was going to everyone every time we saw them. They would only hear the story once, but we found ourselves reliving the same painful experiences over and over and over again. Then we tried sharing our experience in a private group on social media, hoping that we could keep people updated without having to explain things repeatedly.

When we started our third year of IVF treatment, we decided we wanted to share our story online, hoping to help other people going through the same thing. We had become more comfortable with our infertility, and it felt empowering to share our story. That was when we started making YouTube videos and sharing on our social media accounts.

Go to www.InfertilityMan.com/MansGuide to follow our fertility journey.

When we started transferring embryos, we felt the need to become intensely private again, so we simply stopped sharing. It just felt right to keep this part just between the two of us again.

The message here is that you can design your own plan for your privacy and you are allowed to change your mind at different points on your journey. Do what works best for you. You get to decide what the world knows about and you can change your approach at any moment.

Until recently, very few people discussed infertility and reproductive loss, therefore people do not have a socially accepted script to follow. They might even say something with the best of intentions but it just ends up making you feel worse. In fact, it might be the case that someone responds to you with their very best version of empathy and sensitivity, and it still feels like that person said or did the wrong things. For a time, it might feel like nothing others can say will comfort you.

Let go of your expectations for people to be considerate or say the right things. You may need to explain to family, friends and work colleagues how you would like to be supported. Perhaps you would prefer that they don't ask you questions and you will come to them with any news.

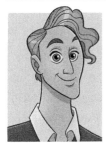

*There are people in my life who I really expected to be a lot more supportive, and they weren't. Some people just found it all way too intimidating and just pulled right back, they couldn't cope with it. Like my brother... just nothing from him... ever. And conversely, there were people in my life who I never expected to be particularly supportive who were incredible. - **Ted***

Unhappiness comes when expectation doesn't equal your reality. Your family and friends can never truly understand how you are feeling, and thank goodness. You wouldn't wish this on anyone else – it's a good thing that they don't know what this feels like.

Sometimes your family members will have to deal with their own feelings of loss about your infertility. Family and friends might have a perceived idea in their heads about the role they will play in your potential children's lives, so your infertility can be a challenge for them to process. The most important thing for you to realise is that you are not responsible for their feelings or reaction to your diagnosis. You hear of couples feeling so guilty that their loved ones are upset that the couple spends more time comforting them than looking after themselves.

In the end, how you share about your difficulties in building your family is totally up to you. If you are seeking a certain type of support, you might need to describe exactly what you need and not expect people to read your mind. They can't.

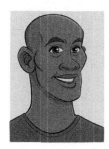

The first year, we didn't really share too much. We were in a bubble, particularly after that first miscarriage. We didn't want to put ourselves through it again, having to tell people about losing the baby. When we were pregnant the second time we didn't tell people the news and then of course we lost that one too. Over time, we learnt to seek out the support that worked for us, we told the people who could understand to some degree. And that helped a lot in the end. - Jaydyn

MANAGING YOUR PROFESSIONALS

Prepare your Support Crew by finding the medical professionals and complementary therapists you want on your side. It is a simple fact that no one can care about your own health and fertility as much as you do. Nor should they – your body and your family is most important to you. Doctors and nurses are caring and intelligent people, but they have potentially hundreds of patients. Though you should be able to expect good service, you won't always get it. You must account for human error and your fertility treatment is far too important to leave to chance.

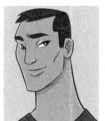

The doctors don't have all the answers.
They don't even know all the questions.
- Leigh

Being your own advocate means asking for what you need while respecting the needs of others. Self-advocacy is asking for what you need in a direct, respectful manner, and this skill is vital when interacting with medical professionals. Be an active participant in your own medical journey and advocate for yourself with your doctors, nurses and anyone else you choose to help with your infertility.

FROM LAURA

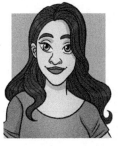

I was on my third or fourth cycle for another IVF egg retrieval. As I hadn't been having a lot of luck with finding eggs in my previous retrievals, my doctor wanted to do a Day 2 ultrasound and blood tests, just to make sure things looked ok at the start of my cycle. The protocol I had been given said that I should inject myself in the morning with a follicle stimulating hormone so I did that at about 7:30 am and then headed into the fertility clinic for my ultrasound and blood test at around 9 am.

I was 36 years old. I had good AMH and FSH levels and I had retrieved a few eggs in previous cycles. I was pretty confident that the cycle would go fairly well. I was hoping to get a few (or hopefully a lot) of eggs for the freezer.

Later that day, I got a phone call from the nurse. She told me that my FSH was extremely high and I was going into early menopause. My cycle was cancelled and I should stop all of my injections. This seemed strange to me based on my previous cycles, but the nurse was adamant.

If this was true, I would never be able to conceive a child. If I stopped the injections that night, it would screw up the cycle completely. In my somewhat hysterical state (remember, I already had some extra hormones in me), my first thought was to call Jon. Being the level-headed one of the two of us, Jon suggested we should probably listen to the nurse, stop the injections and talk to our doctor when we had the chance.

I went home and continued to wrestle with the news in my mind. Pacing back and forth, I just couldn't shake the feeling that this didn't seem right. How could things go from being ok last month to no good at all this month? My body couldn't have entered menopause that quickly. I was still having normal periods...how could this be?

We have always been taught to listen to our doctors. They are incredibly intelligent and well-trained people. If a medical test result comes back and says something is wrong, you can't deny it.

By the time Jon got home from work, I was pretty upset – talk about having to deal with an avalanche of emotions as soon as he walked in the door! He gave me a big hug, helped to calm me down, and together we made a proactive decision.

They booked me in for a special appointment to see my doctor on Monday. It was Friday, so I would have to wait all weekend. We decided that until we spoke with our doctor face-to-face and saw the test results with our own eyes, we would continue with the injections and the cycle as prescribed. We knew it wouldn't do me any harm and if there was any hope of continuing the cycle; we wanted to try.

As I had my injections that evening, I had tears streaming down my face. I bargained with the universe, "Please don't let this be my last injection!" I said to Jon, "Please don't let this be my last injection." After months of dreading my injections and feeling sick and miserable about fertility treatment, I was begging, please, don't let this be the end of our journey with IVF.

On the Monday morning (after repeating the whole emotional injection experience several more times) Jon and I went to the fertility clinic to meet with our doctor. We were dreading the appointment because we already knew what we were expecting to hear. Normally the clinic runs pretty much on time but this morning (of course) they were over an hour behind. We sat there waiting for what seemed like an eternity.

When my name was finally called, my heart leapt into my throat. I didn't want to go in because I didn't want to hear this news. My doctor began to tell us in a very caring way that my test results showed a very high FSH level and that I was likely going into early menopause. Inside my head voices were screaming "It's not true, I'm sure this isn't true for me!" but I tried to listen patiently and absorb what he was saying. I tried to accept it. I leaned over just to double check that the paperwork was correct and saw my name on the paper.

I thought I would try one more thing to prove that these results were incorrect and that this couldn't be happening to me. I asked my doctor, "Is there any chance that the injection that I took the morning of my blood test could alter the results?"

There was a moment of silence. The doctor said, "Oh, did you take your injection that morning?"

"Yes."

My doctor exclaimed, "Oh well, don't worry about any of this, you're fine, your FSH was only elevated because of the meds!"

The three of us looked at each other in shock. I burst out laughing and crying at the same time. I repeated the information in order to confirm it (another trick for making sure you understand the medical professionals). "So, we're fine, I'm not going into early menopause, we can continue with the cycle, IVF could still work for us?"

I had never felt so much relief. Maybe some women (who were more experienced with IVF than I was at the time) would have realised right away where the mistake had been made. I had just trusted that my doctor had told me the correct times to take my injections and that the nurses would take that into account when reading the blood test results. We learned a valuable lesson that day. Doctors and nurses can make mistakes. Human error is part of this process. No one will ever pay as much attention to your health and your fertility as you will.

As we walked out of the office and into the busy waiting area, my doctor exclaimed, "You guys should write a book!" We were laughing (and crying) *and everyone sitting in the waiting room was looking at us inquisitively, wondering what on earth had just happened in there. The receptionist even asked us if we were happy to share. (Incidentally, we did share a lot, in the following days with everyone in the clinic. We wanted to make sure this never happened to any other patients).*

Thank goodness I asked questions. Thank goodness we continued with our cycle and didn't stop taking the injections. Thank goodness we didn't just accept the diagnosis and walk out of the clinic, forever giving up on the idea that I could ever get pregnant.

That evening, I had never been more grateful to take my injections, I was just so grateful that I was still in the game. Even though we needed IVF to conceive, we are still very lucky to have that option. Many people don't. I never looked at my injections the same way again.

Ensure you get the best medical care

If you look at any of the online fertility forums, you will often see people who are frustrated with the medical care they are receiving. You hear stories of doctors not remembering important details, nurses making mistakes and appointments running hours late. It's understandable that patients are sometimes upset. Fertility treatment costs a lot, and when something is expensive we expect it to be good. People talk about venting their frustrations to receptionists, writing angry emails and having heated phone conversations.

Infertility treatment is already a difficult process. You have a right to be annoyed at anything that makes it harder. We felt this way occasionally too, until we realised that getting angry would not help us get better treatment and more attention from our doctor. Fertility clinics have hundreds of patients, how can you get the personalised care that you deserve? We realised that being a memorable patient would work much better than getting frustrated and complaining. Being friendly and polite to the busy staff would work better than being unkind.

Here are some ways to participate in your treatment and be a memorable patient:

▶ Prepare for your appointments. Come in with a written list of topics you want to discuss.
▶ Write notes or ask to record audio of your appointments to help you remember details.
▶ Make friends with the doctors and nurses.
▶ Remember the nurses' and receptionists' names, write them down if that helps.
▶ Build a personal relationship with the medical staff, ask about their families, talk about the rugby and find out what you have in common.
▶ Be respectful. You catch more bees with honey.
▶ Give little appropriate gifts to your medical team, even early in your relationship.
▶ Be forgiving, for example, when appointments are running late.
▶ Ask that just one nurse oversees your case, especially if it is a really big clinic.
▶ Share your story online. This option is not for everyone, but sometimes having people following your journey online can make your doctor just a little more aware of your case. However, only speak positively about your fertility clinic online, bring any negative concerns to them directly.

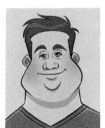

Once we moved to our new doctor, her care was unbelievable. She's such an amazing doctor, even receiving bad news from her felt really good, like it was taking us a step closer to finding the answer. - Blake

You're the Boss

Your fertility treatment is like a business and you are the project manager. You are in charge, with your partner, if you have one. Any person who works on your fertility project can be hired or fired at any moment. You can replace them at any time and try out someone new. You can see another doctor and get a second opinion. If it's not working, you have the power to change it.

Even family and friends can be temporarily or permanently removed from your fertility support crew. They will still remain your family and friends, but they no longer get to advise on fertility issues. You might even find acquaintances who surprise you, they may not be very close to you at the start of your fertility journey, but it turns out they understand better than your usual confidants.

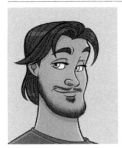 *It is really amazing how many people have been through IVF. It's remarkable, I told someone at work and suddenly they say, 'Oh Mark from accounts went through that'... so you chat to him and he ends up being the most amazing support. As soon as you open up, bang! There really is a plethora of people who have been through it.* **- Jamie**

At any time, you can take breaks from confiding in the people who aren't able to support you. You can choose to ignore people who make insensitive comments. Set up the boundaries that are necessary to protect your heart and ensure you receive the best care. Be kind and gentle in your approach, but in the end, your experience right now is too challenging to tiptoe around, concerned about hurting people's feelings. No one has the right to be part of your fertility journey. It's a privilege to be involved and you get to choose who you trust to be in your inner circle.

BABY MAKING TEAM

YOUR SUPPORT CREW

COMPLEMENTARY

ACUPUNCTURIST

MASSAGE THERAPIST

NUTRITIONIST

COUNSELLOR

CHIROPRACTOR

INFORMATIONAL

BOOKS

ONLINE RESOURCES

FERTILITY
BLOGGER

SOCIAL

FAMILY

FRIENDS

WORK COLLEAGUES

KIND
STRANGERS

MEDICAL

DOCTOR

UROLOGIST

FERTILITY CLINIC

ANAESTHETIST

NURSES

PEOPLE TEMPORARILY OR PERMANENTLY REMOVED FROM SUPPORT CREW

FERTILITY
INFLUENCER

PRACTITIONER OF
BIZARRE TREATMENTS

PREGNANT SISTER WHO
DOESN'T UNDERSTAND

AUNT WHO SAYS
INSENSITIVE THINGS

THE DOCTOR WHO
DIDN'T LISTEN TO YOU

BABY-MAKING MEET UP

Support Crew

- ▶ Who do you need to tell that you are trying to conceive or that you are seeking fertility treatment?
- ▶ Who will be on your support crew?
- ▶ Who has provided you with helpful, non-judgemental support in the past?
- ▶ How and when will you tell them?
- ▶ How can you describe and request the support that you would like from them?
- ▶ What is important to keep private?
- ▶ Who do you agree not to tell?
- ▶ Who do you need to gently remove from your support crew?
- ▶ What do you hope to achieve by telling people and how can you be clear about your needs?
- ▶ Will you tell your employer or colleagues about your fertility treatment?
- ▶ Which medical professionals and complementary therapists will you choose to support you?
- ▶ How can you be a memorable patient?

Draw an organisational chart of all the people who will support you during your fertility treatment, including medical professionals, complementary therapists, friends and family.

See the Baby-Making Meet Up videos and download a workbook at www.InfertilityMan.com/MansGuide

YOUR RELATIONSHIP

If you have a partner, your relationship with them is most important, as you navigate infertility. You will learn so much about yourself, your partner, and your relationship. Even if your relationship is super solid, you should still consider counselling at this challenging time. It is too much to manage with just the two of you, and there are professionals who can support you.

There are several ways that infertility puts a strain on relationships.

▶ **Stress on your sexual relationship**
What starts out as a sexy whisper of "Let's make a baby" over time can become a real drag and the last thing you want to think about. Strain on your sexual relationship is common in couples struggling with infertility, especially if they are timing intercourse, hoping to conceive a baby.

▶ **Disagreements about telling other people**
Often one partner is ready to seek advice from a doctor, while the other still hopes that it will happen naturally next month. This can lead to conflict and frustration.

▶ **Fears of being left because of infertility**
When you are diagnosed as infertile, it may bring up fears that your partner will leave to be with someone who can easily conceive.

▶ **Disagreement about telling other people**
Infertility can bring up feelings of embarrassment or shame. One partner may want to tell friends and family to seek support, whereas the other may prefer to keep it a secret. They may feel that infertility is too private a topic to share.

► **Resentment**

Resentment can form when only one partner is diagnosed with infertility or when one must endure more of the fertility treatment. Unresolved feelings of guilt or blame can lead to tension.

► **Financial strain**

It's no secret that infertility can wreak havoc on finances. Arguments about money are not unique to infertile couples, however, because fertility treatment can be very expensive, the pressure can be even more intense. IVF and medical costs can lead to financial stress that follows you for quite some time, with no guarantee of conceiving a child. Disagreements can arise from differences of opinion on how to spend money on treatment, whether and how to borrow money, whether to ask friends and family for assistance, and when to stop.

► **Difference of opinion on how to proceed**

Couples may experience tension because they have different ideas on how to move forward. Disagreements may be about debt and medical bills, or the emotional and physical discomfort of continuing with the treatments themselves. Couples may quarrel over whether to take temporary breaks or whether to move on for good. They may disagree on whether to pursue other paths to parenthood or to live a child-free life.

► **Misunderstandings**

Everyone copes with stress differently. These differences can lead to misunderstandings. For example, one partner may be accused of 'not caring enough' if their coping style is more subdued. Alternatively, the other partner may be charged with 'overreacting'.

THE TICKING OF THE CLOCK

Generally, the differences in how men and women respond to infertility can be traced back to biology. It is a simple physiological fact that women have fewer fertile years than men. This creates a difference in their sense of timing. Every day, every year, every birthday and every failed cycle can feel like she is running out of time.

One of the best ways you can support your partner is by being aware and responsive to her timeline. You may feel less urgency than her in lining up fertility related engagements. A wait to get a doctor's appointment may not feel like a big deal to you, but it might feel like a very painful delay to her. Not getting the paperwork done before her next period in order to begin an IVF cycle can feel to her like another wasted month.

Understand that her timeline is different from yours and be responsive. If she asks you to do something, realise that she may be feeling an incredible time pressure and do it as promptly as possible.

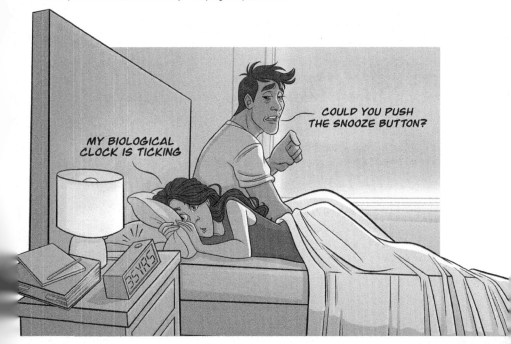

Surviving the Storm

A 2014 study of almost 50,000 Danish women found that women who don't have a child after fertility treatment are three times more likely to divorce or end cohabitation with their partner than those who do.

A later study in 2017 did not find that couples undertaking assisted reproductive therapy were more likely to separate than the general population. The author of the study, Dr Mariana Martins from the Faculty of Psychology at the University of Porto, Portugal said, "We also know that despite all the strain that infertility can bring, going through ART can actually bring benefit to a couple's relationship, because it forces them to improve communication and coping strategies."

So it is not infertility or IVF that dictates whether your relationship will survive, but rather how you treat each other while you are going through it. Infertility is not forever. You may or may not have children one day, but you won't be struggling to conceive forever. Your relationship can survive this tough but temporary challenge. In fact, you might come out the other side even stronger.

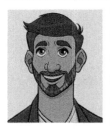

*To be honest, I'm probably not the best source of information on how to deal with it all. Not because I'm a closed book, I'm not a 'grunty' man who shows no emotions. I take after my father, his theory is, worry about something when there is something to worry about. My priority was always to look after her. And so, I guess my coping mechanism was knowing that I was being the best possible support for my wife that I could be. - **Lesley**

STOP TRYING TO FIX IT!

A common dilemma is when one person in a couple is upset about something (in your case, most likely infertility) and looking for emotional support from their partner, but the other person only wants to try to solve the problem. The support seeking person gets upset because they feel their partner has not listened. The problem-solving partner is confused and frustrated because they don't understand why their partner simply won't take their advice to fix things. Often this occurs in a gendered way. Stereotypically, it's the woman who wants emotional support and the man who wants to solve the problem.

Masculine people are often wired to protect and provide. And that is why infertility sucks. We can't protect our partner from the pain and frustration that comes along with wanting children and struggling to have them, and we can't provide the very thing that would take all the hurt away. When men can't solve a problem, we tend to put it out of our minds until such time that we can solve it. We can't do anything about it right now, so why think about it?

Feminine people are often wired to communicate and connect through sharing their stories and challenges. They want to be heard and understood. It is this connecting that makes them feel better, rather than the actual solving of their problem.

These two different approaches can cause difficulties. One partner wants to connect and feel their pain surrounding infertility while the other is frustrated by them constantly bringing it up, as they can't immediately solve the problem. Any solutions they offer seem to upset their partner, rather than bring them the peace they seek.

Infertility is an incredibly difficult problem that can take years to solve. Having this dynamic in your relationship in an ongoing way could really cause problems. It is so important to bring some awareness to your behaviour so that you can both feel heard and understood.

BEING PRESENT

You don't need to have all the answers or be able to immediately fix your fertility woes. This is good news because you won't be able to – infertility is too large a problem to be solved on your own. It can sometimes take months and even years to resolve. When your partner is sharing her emotions with you regarding your situation, all you need to do is to be present.

Being present means actively listening and connecting. That is often as simple as listening while making comforting sounds or comments and without offering solutions.

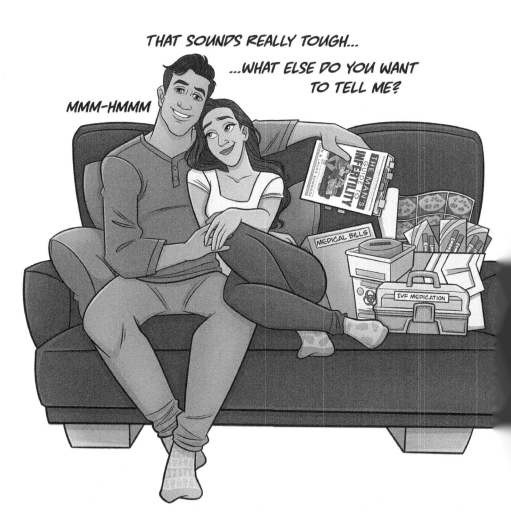

VENTING

The female brain functions a little differently from yours. Women's brains have more connectivity between the left hemisphere, which is more analytical, and the right hemisphere, which is more creative and intuitive. Women's brains generally can read social situations with far more complexity than us guys can, because their brains are wired differently. Generally, men are more 'single focused'. We like to focus on one thing at a time. Women, on the other hand, have what has been called 'diffused awareness'. They can process more things simultaneously and focus on many things at once. Her brain is a wide-angled lens. She is hyper aware of anything related to pregnancy or babies, resulting in the perfect recipe for feeling like crap. This means that she really is thinking and feeling about infertility ALL. THE. TIME. She is wired to have infertility at least at the back of her mind, all the time. It may mean she is wired for upset and perhaps poor mental health.

Masculine energy is generally about 'letting go' – everything we do is about achieving the goal and then letting go, releasing and relaxing. Feminine energy is the opposite. Throughout her day she is collecting and gathering, ending up with a mind full of thoughts, ideas and worries. Especially when it comes to fertility. She notices every pregnant woman, every happy family, and every insensitive comment. By the time she comes back to you, she is carrying a heavy mental load.

This is where the concept of 'venting' can be helpful. You hold out a metaphorical rubbish bin and allow her to vent out all the difficult thoughts and feelings into it. Your job is not to solve her problems or argue with her that things are not as bad as she thinks. Your job is to hold out that metaphorical bin and allow her to empty herself of all the stressful emotions. She may say things that seem over the top or even ridiculously negative, but you just stay with her and allow her to process these feelings. And when you think she is finished, you can ask her this question: "Is there anything else you want to share with me?"

This will either unleash another tirade of emotion about how difficult infertility is to live with, or you will notice a change in her. Look out for the change. If she has shared with you all her emotions and she has felt heard, she will reach a point where she can also relax and let go. She will feel that you have understood her and lightened her mental load.

Occasionally, your partner may need to vent to someone else, a friend, a sister or her mother, for example. She might even want to vent her frustration about you or share information that you consider to be private. Do your best to be understanding and realise that she may process her emotions differently to you.

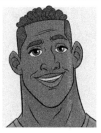

I think the most difficult thing for me was coping with my wife's ups and downs and seeing the person I love more than anybody else, my absolute soul mate, my rock, going through the traumas that she went through. That was the thing that was distressing. I can deal with it personally, I can deal with it when it is happening to me, but watching her at times was so traumatic. That was the hard stuff. - Damien

LOVE LANGUAGES

One of the common relationship issues people face is the struggle to communicate. On a deeper level, it is challenging to show your partner love and to have them feel that love.

In his landmark book *The 5 Love Languages*, Dr Gary Chapman presents the idea that we all communicate and understand love through five languages.

► **Words of Affirmation**
This love language is about expressing affection through spoken words, praise, or appreciation. For a couple going through infertility this could look like thanking her for all the injections she is taking, telling her what a great job she is doing in managing all the IVF paperwork, complimenting her on her bravery, leaving a cute note in her medicine bag, telling her she looks hot in a hospital gown or sending a text message to wish her luck at her doctor's appointment.

► **Quality Time**
Love and affection are expressed through this love language by giving her your undivided attention. Notice that it is called quality time and not quantity time – you don't need hours and hours to show love in this way. For fertility warriors this can be as simple as being 100 percent present for baby-making conversations, attending doctor's appointments and making them fun, giving good eye contact during uncomfortable medical procedures and actively connecting and being with her while she is recovering from surgery.

► **Physical Touch**
A person with this love language feels loved through physical affection. In terms of infertility, this could mean holding her hand during a difficult moment at a baby shower, giving her a back rub while she is feeling unwell due to hormone injections, or cuddling on the couch after a failed IVF cycle.

► Acts of Service

When your partner's primary love language is acts of service, she will feel loved and appreciated when you do nice things for her. During the period of your life when you are trying to conceive this could mean helpful acts such as going to the pharmacy to pick up her IVF drugs, setting alarms to remind you when it is time for injections and preparing the medications or picking her up from the hospital. Taking care of day-to-day household chores so that she can focus on the arduous tasks associated with fertility treatment would also be extremely well-received.

► Gifts

To a person whose love language is receiving gifts, receiving presents is a symbol of love and affection. They treasure not only the gift itself but also the time and effort put into it. They don't necessarily expect large or expensive gifts, it is the thought that counts. In the fertility world, gifts could be related to their medical procedures, good luck charms on transfer day or thoughtful presents during difficult times.

We all feel and express love differently. It's unlikely that you and your partner value the same love languages equally. The way you show love to your partner and the way you receive love may be different. Consequently, putting some thought into which love languages you and your partner value most could significantly improve your communication and the way you both feel within your relationship. We all enjoy variety, so even though your partner may favour one love language, you can still mix it up and show love in a range of different ways.

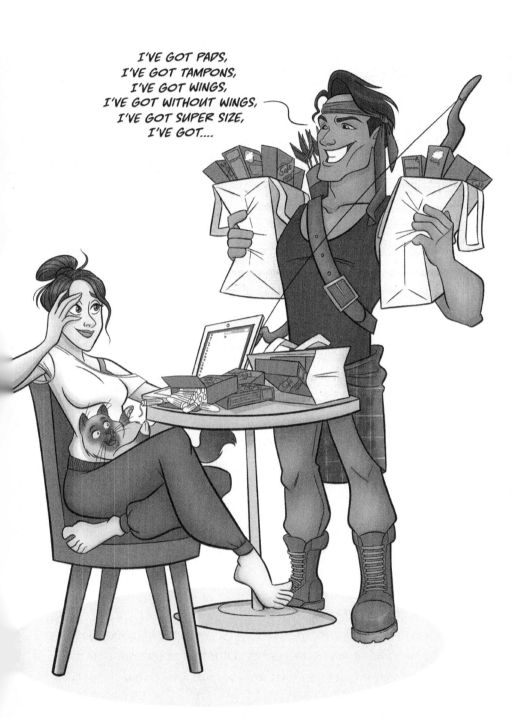

FROM LAURA

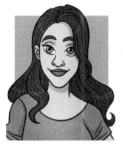 *During my IVF cycles, I felt sick. I was bloated and in pain and I had to give myself injections three times a day… which was not fun. Thankfully, my calmer and more practical partner Jon was on hand to help. Turns out he's more emotionally balanced than me and much better in difficult situations. I suppose that is why he is a paramedic. On many occasions during my IVF cycles, I felt like I was in an emergency situation… turns out, I was not – it just felt that way. Trust me when I say that your role as partner in this fertility process is more important than you may realise. Little things you do to help may not feel like a lot to you, but they make a lot of difference.*

Here is how Jon helped me:

1. He asked me if I was ok and if I said I wasn't, he helped me to realise that I really was ok.
Being on fertility medication can be a rollercoaster of emotions. I felt excited, but scared and sad. I felt physically sick. I was terrified about what the outcome of our IVF treatment would be, but also happy that we were making progress. And tired, I felt so very tired. It was very confusing.

Jon listened to my feelings, but also didn't allow me to wallow in them and helped me find ways to move forward.

2. He encouraged me to take time out.
I was trying to work and keep doing everything I had been doing before, but my body just wouldn't allow me to do that. He gave me permission to take breaks and have afternoon naps, in a way that I wasn't really giving myself.

3. *He took charge of the housework.*

If your partner is anything like me, she likes to limit the clutter and mess and can be pedantic about housework. Overflowing laundry baskets and sinks full of dishes make me feel like crap.

In my uncomfortable and hormonal state, managing housework while maturing lots of eggs in my ovaries felt insurmountable. That's when Jon stepped up.

He also likes the house to be clean, so he did a lot more to take on my share of the cleaning. He did all the mundane chores. He'd unload the dishwasher, wipe down the bench tops and put on a load of washing.

If there was anything I'd asked him to do, it would get done. And most of the time, I didn't have to ask.

4. *He bought groceries.*

I really wanted to eat healthy food during my IVF cycles, but sometimes the thought of getting out of the house to buy groceries was just too much. So Jon made sure we had a well-stocked fridge and pantry. Sometimes I would feel so sick that I could only eat certain things, so he would pick up anything extra that I needed.

5. *He didn't bother me for intimacy.*

Sorry guys, you know where this is going and, yes, I know it's tough. But when Jon understood my reluctance for intimacy, I couldn't have loved him more. I still appreciated him initiating physical touch and letting me know he was attracted to me, but when I showed I wasn't feeling up to it, he never made it a big deal.

My ovaries were the size of golf balls for months at a time and my stomach was bloated and painful to touch. And I also just felt pretty bad about myself. Sex was sometimes the last thing I felt like doing.

All the missed opportunities were made up when I was feeling healthy again in between IVF cycles. His understanding and kindness made me want to be intimate with him even more.

6. He always had faith in me.

Doing 15 IVF cycles was the hardest thing I have ever done. Physically, mentally, and emotionally, it was like a marathon. There were many times when I felt like I wasn't going to make it. Every time we experienced a setback or received bad news, I really took it to heart. I felt like a lot of the troubles we had were my fault, as I just couldn't get my body to do what I thought it was supposed to do.

Jon always had faith in me. When I didn't respond to IVF medications and thought I would never be able to have a baby, he showed me the reality of our situation with a bit of hope thrown in. From day one, he had my back. He convinced me I was doing a great job and supported me with every decision. Without his support, I wouldn't have had the confidence to keep going and without his help, I wouldn't have ever made it all the way.

So, while as men, you may feel a little sidelined during some parts of fertility treatment, please know that you're still a key player in this game. Every little thing you do to help is so special to us... even if we're so hormonal we forget to say thanks!

FROM JON

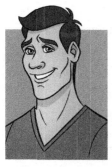

It was such a challenge for me to watch my beautiful lady go through the turmoil and torment of the IVF process. Injection after injection, bruising, tears, bloating. All you can do is sit back and be in awe of your partner. She is doing this so you both have a shot at conceiving a child and it is by no means a walk in the park. Worship the ground she walks on, treat her as your number one responsibility and make this process as smooth as it can possibly be for her. If she wants a cuddle, give her a cuddle. If she wants a tea, make her tea. Be with her and listen to her. You do not need to fix anything, she just wants to be heard by you. And most of all, do the injections for her if she would like you to. Just being there with her and sending your positive energy helps her to feel supported and at the end of the day, that is what you want for her. Make sure she knows she can depend on you, no matter what.

Unconditional

Love is unconditional. It works best when people come to a relationship intending to give rather than receive. If you want something from your partner, the first thing you should do is to give it unconditionally. Truly unconditionally, with no expectation of getting it back. If you want your partner to be more supportive during infertility, then start by being more supportive of them. If you don't want someone nagging you or trying to change you, then don't nag or try to change someone else. If you want less judgment, then stop being judgmental. If you want more kindness and attention, be kind and attentive.

Taking care of your relationship will not only help you navigate the challenging world of infertility but also to set up behaviours and habits that will be invaluable to you in your life. When faced with a challenge like infertility, you can find untapped reserves of strength within yourself. Many couples even find that going through this experience together strengthens their relationship and they come out even better on the other side.

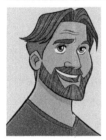

*Infertility breaks some people, it makes others. We're fortunate that on the other side of it, we're now invincible. - **Josh***

BABY-MAKING MEET UP

Over a nice meal, have a chat about how you can prioritise your relationship as you go through this challenging time of infertility.

► Ask her if there is anything she would like to share with you.

► Listen without trying to solve her problem. Then ask her, "Is there anything else?"

► Talk about how you can support each other even better as you go through your fertility treatments.

► What are her top two love languages?

► What are yours?

► Is there a difference between how you both give and receive love?

See the Baby-Making Meet Up videos and download a workbook at www.InfertilityMan.com/MansGuide

INTERACTING WITH THE WORLD

Imagine waking up every day feeling like something is bothering you. What is it again? Oh yes, it's the fact that you don't have a child, you may never have a child and you may have to rethink your whole life's purpose and everything you envisioned for your future. That is a lot to have constantly in the back of your mind every day. At the same time, you are attempting to have a normal life, congratulating everyone around you on their pregnancies, their births, their child's birthday, their second pregnancy, their second birth, their third pregnancy, and so on. You are most likely at an age where it seems like everyone you know is having children, so there is really no escaping it. Your partner may be particularly aware of this. Suddenly, everywhere she looks, there are pregnant women and children. It's not just family and friends. Suddenly, it seems like everyone is growing their families; celebrities, co-workers, people on the street, women on trains to whom she has to give up her seat while envying their rounded tummies.

The reticular activating system (RAS) is a bundle of nerves at our brainstem that filters out unnecessary information so the important stuff gets through. It's the reason when you buy a specific type of new car, you suddenly see that model of car everywhere. It's why you can tune out a crowd full of talking people, yet immediately snap to attention when someone says your name. When you are focused on becoming pregnant, suddenly it feels like pregnancies surround you. They were always there before, but you notice them now more than ever. It's almost like you put on special goggles programmed to show you everything to do with pregnancy, babies and fertility. It can become tiresome to constantly be reminded of the one thing that is currently beyond your reach.

The feeling that everyone around you is moving forward and building their families while you cannot brings up unwanted feelings of envy. In addition, many people who are experiencing infertility also describe another round of guilt because they feel jealous. They think,

'I'm not a person who feels jealous of other people's happiness! That is mean-spirited. Why can't I feel happy for them? I should want the best for other people, so why am I so upset?'

FROM LAURA

I was at work one day and in the middle of an IVF cycle. The medications were really affecting me. My ovaries were very swollen and my tummy hurt quite a lot. I was aching and tired.

I hadn't told anyone at work that we were doing IVF. It didn't feel like the right thing to do, and I knew I was still a long way off from being pregnant. One reason I had told no one was because several of the women I worked with were pregnant. I didn't want to put a dampener on their happiness. I wanted them to be able to talk about their pregnancies without having to worry about me.

I had just returned from giving myself an injection in the public bathroom stall. It had bled quite a lot and I almost got blood on my clothes, so I was frazzled. Two pregnant colleagues were standing nearby when we received a delivery of boxes. They looked at me, expecting that I would be the one to carry the boxes to the storeroom. My workmates were pregnant, so of course, they shouldn't do it. I couldn't think of a reason that I could tell them why I probably shouldn't be lifting either, even though my ovaries felt like they would pop.

As I put my head down and began slowly moving the heavy boxes, I thought to myself, 'wow, this is the real everyday experience of infertility. Suffering in silence, just wishing that you could share happier news. Always stepping aside to take care of pregnant people and celebrating their milestones as they grow their families and keeping your own pain to yourself.'

Turn it around

It is so difficult, but try not to compare your situation with others. We can never truly know what someone else has lived through. It may look like a social media photo of perfection, but we all know life is not like that. Maybe they struggled to conceive too, maybe they have difficulties in their relationship or maybe they are struggling with being a parent or with postnatal depression.

Every time you see something pregnancy related think in your head, *It's so wonderful that...* and finish the sentence with a positive answer.

- ► It's so wonderful that they could get pregnant easily. I wouldn't want them to experience infertility.
- ► It's so wonderful that women her age can get pregnant. Maybe that will happen to us too.
- ► It's so wonderful that I care enough to feel upset about this. It shows that I really care about having a baby and makes me even more determined and resilient.

It is possible to feel happy for someone else while feeling terribly sad for yourself. It's even ok not to feel happy for them at all, as long as you don't behave in a way that would hurt anyone else. These feelings can be confusing, so it is important to understand that you can feel two opposite feelings at the same time. Acknowledge these competing emotions and understand that whatever you or your partner is feeling, it's ok. It is perfectly reasonable given the circumstances. Be kind to yourself and your partner. Fighting with your own emotions is exhausting and unhelpful. It is ok to feel sadness for your situation while at the same time celebrating someone else's joy.

Share these thoughts and feelings with your baby-making team, or with a counsellor. It is important to reconcile conflicting emotions, so discussing them with a non-judgemental external person can help.

Tip: Be sensitive when you break joyful news about someone else's pregnancy to your partner. And *always* prepare her, if you happen to hear about a new pregnancy before she does. Don't let her be blindsided by a pregnancy announcement. If this means violating someone else's trust and sharing their secret, then do it. Every time someone else gets pregnant, her first thought is going to be that she wishes it were her. She may not be able to mask that emotion, which will not feel great for the pregnant friend either. Tell her in private, give her a chance to brace herself and have time to come to terms with it. She can always act surprised and hopefully she can seem happy if she has had a chance to prepare.

THE THINGS PEOPLE SAY

Have you experienced the painful cringe that makes your heart beat a little faster when someone asks if you have kids? The awkward pause that makes you want to scream when someone asks if you plan to have babies soon. The immediate eye-roll that is followed by anger when someone tells you how lucky you are to be able to sleep because you don't have any children. Or if you already have a child, they ask when you are going to give them a sibling. The fake laugh you force while your soul secretly crushes when someone complains about their pregnancy or 'mum life' to you.

When you share with people that you are struggling to conceive, their comments can be insensitive.

► My friend suffered from infertility for 12 years before finally becoming a parent!
► Have you tried this or that?
► Ugh, you can have one of my kids!
► Oh you're lucky, having kids is such hard work.
► I hated being pregnant.
► You should just adopt!
► Just stop trying, then you'll get pregnant.
► I wish I had your problem! All my husband has to do is look at me and I get pregnant.
► You just need to trust. God/The Universe will send you a child in time.
► Maybe you just weren't meant to have kids.
► Just relax!

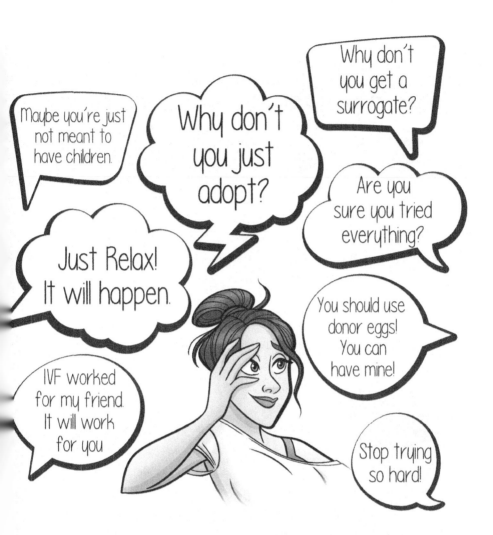

Infertility means pretending you're ok in the eyes of the public when all you want to do is curl up in a ball and cry. It just sucks. As awareness grows around infertility and pregnancy loss, hopefully we are moving towards becoming a more compassionate society. Unfortunately, people will always behave in a way that reflects their level of consciousness and you can't change that. Some days you might feel resilient enough to educate them about what you are going through and other days you will need to protect your own heart and not engage in the conversation. Just smile and nod and get away from them as soon as you can!

In the Mindsets of Infertility, fertile people will always be in Mindset Number 1.

THE 7 MINDSETS OF INFERTILITY

1	2	3	4	5	6	7
BELIEVING YOU CAN CONCEIVE NATURALLY	BELIEVING YOU CAN CONCEIVE WITH FERTILITY TREATMENT	CHOOSING TO USE DONOR EGGS, SPERM OR EMBRYOS	CONFIDENT THAT YOU CAN CARRY A PREGNANCY TO TERM	CHOOSING TO ENGAGE A SURROGATE OR GESTATIONAL CARRIER	EXPLORING OTHER PARENTING PATHWAYS LIKE ADOPTION	COMING TO TERMS WITH BEING CHILDLESS

This makes it difficult for them to understand what it feels like to be in any other position, which is why they can say insensitive things. Most of the time, they do not intend to be unkind.

Although it sucks, at least you can notice that you are becoming more compassionate towards people through your experiences.

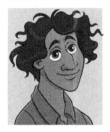

I had testicular cancer and don't produce sperm... and no sperm comes out due to retrograde ejaculation (when semen enters the bladder instead of emerging through the penis). People keep telling us stories about how someone they knew got pregnant after trying for so long and that we should 'just relax' because when we least expect it, it will happen. I mean, well done to those people, but it's impossible that will happen in our situation. **- David**

FEELING INFERTILE AT GATHERINGS

Celebrations, parties and family gatherings can be difficult when you're trying to conceive. You may find yourself surrounded by babies and children while being bombarded with uncomfortable questions and conversations.

While you are going through the challenging experience of infertility, your most important responsibility is to take care of yourself and your partner. It is imperative for you to pay attention to your partner's needs at this time and not, for example, forget about them in favour of your mother, your father, your sister, your brother or your best friend.

You might want to surround yourselves with family members or you might not. You might want to go to parties, baby showers and celebrations or you might not. Or she might not. You might think that you want to go and then change your mind at the last minute. Be gentle with yourself and each other. Don't force yourself to attend uncomfortable gatherings, especially if you are not going to add positive energy to the event. It is vital to take care of yourself.

If you decide to go, remember that the party is about the people being celebrated and you will need to keep your emotions in check. Interestingly, focusing your attention on someone else's joy might actually make you feel better, even if only momentarily. It is an incredibly generous thing for you to do, and generosity always feels good. So if you are going to go to a baby shower or a child's birthday party, go with your whole heart. Focus on the guests of honour and behave as you would hope others behave if one day you are lucky enough to be celebrating the same milestone.

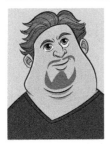

*We didn't really say much to other people, we just held on to each other and battled through it. The hardest part was going to family events. All my cousins have got kids and they would say, 'You guys will be next!' We would think 'That would be f***king nice!' - **Ben***

Have a plan to take care of yourself and your partner.

▶ Do what you can to keep it out of sight and out of mind until the actual event. Sometimes the week leading up can be harder than the actual event. Stay busy, do yoga, meditate, workout, clean. Keep any anxiety to one day rather than an entire week.

▶ If buying a baby gift would be difficult for you, ask someone else to do it on your behalf or contribute money to a group gift.

▶ Do something before the event to get you in the best possible mood, such as a short walk, while you think about how much you care for the people at the party.

▶ Go to the event but for a shorter time. Arrive a little late and leave before it gets to be too much for you.

▶ Find people at the party who don't want kids or aren't interested in kids at this stage of their life. Your conversations will not revolve around pregnancy or baby milestones. Plus, these people are usually awesome and you might momentarily forget where you are.

▶ If someone is socially uneducated and makes comments about when you will have kids, walk away. People should know better than to say things like that these days. Or you may choose to take a moment to gently educate them, but remember, it's not your job to change the world.

▶ Lean on your partner or a friend you trust. Work out a signal between you to let each other know when you need to leave. And then leave together immediately.

- Have another signal so you can connect with each other from across the room as a reminder that you are looking out for each other.
- Don't drink too much.
- Pack tissues in your pocket, just in case.
- Plan something enjoyable for after the party, so you have something fun and distracting to look forward to afterwards. A date night, a massage, a road trip, something to bring you and your partner immediate joy.

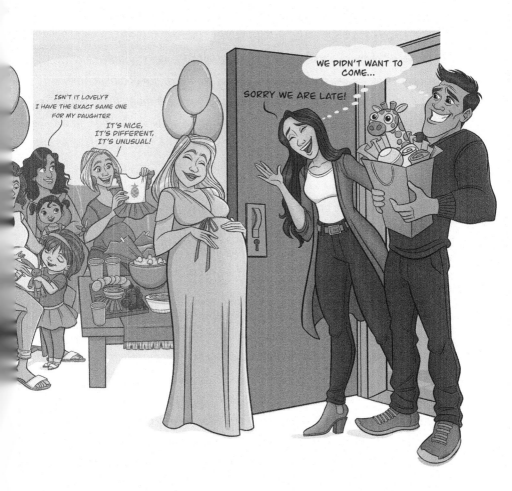

FROM JON

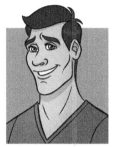

When we were right in the middle of our infertility experience, it seemed that everyone in Laura's life was having babies. Her sisters had three babies during that time and so many of her friends were popping out kids. We were invited to many baby showers and kids' birthday parties – we declined most of the invitations. We decided to only go to events when we felt resilient enough to cope.

We would prepare ourselves beforehand, because even though many people knew we were doing IVF, we didn't want to put a dampener on the celebration. We had lots of strategies to help us through those days. We would have a chat in the morning about how we were feeling and we would look after each other at the party and sometimes we would leave early to do something fun to take our mind off things.

We went to a lovely one-year-old baby's birthday party, right after an IVF cycle that had been cancelled because of poor response. We entered the party with an almost over the top happy energy. We were so focused on making sure that no one pitied us that we overdid it a little, showing that we were fine.

It was such a beautiful celebration, which made it even harder for us knowing that we might never throw a party like that ourselves.

During the speeches, I could see that Laura was struggling a little. I didn't want to do anything to draw attention to us, so I just reached out my foot to touch hers, just to remind her that we were in it together and that I understood how she felt. I saw her shoulders relax and a sad smile spread across her face. Even though it was a tiny gesture, I knew it made all the difference.

NAVIGATING THE ONLINE WORLD

If you type 'infertility' or 'IVF' into a search engine, you will find a vast number of websites, books, blogs, support groups, social media influencers and many people going through the same thing. While not a community anyone takes any joy in joining, there is some comfort in being part of a tribe. Everything we experience these days is mirrored by how we experience it online, and infertility is no different. However, the digital world can have both a positive and negative impact on those experiencing infertility.

Dr Google

When you learn that you have a medical condition that will complicate your plans to become pregnant, it is easy to become immersed in online research. There is a temptation to go online and look up every symptom, treatment and old-fashioned tale, hoping to find the answer to your challenges. Be careful about which online information you trust. Remember that nothing beats professional medical advice that is tailored to your situation, which you can only receive from a qualified person who knows your case.

Social Media

For people experiencing infertility, social media can be a source of great upset or a place to feel connection.

We all know that social media never tells the whole story. People make their lives out to appear better than they actually are. And people post many, many photos of their children. It can be extremely triggering to see photos of your friends' children, as well as pregnancy and birth announcements. If someone online is getting you down, while you may not need to 'unfriend' them, it can help to unfollow that person to make their posts show up less in your feed. You might even need to take breaks from social media to protect your mental health.

Alternatively, while infertility may make a person feel alienated from people in real life, social media can provide community and psychological support. Finding others who are going through similar experiences can help in the realisation that you're not alone and that your feelings are reasonable. Online infertility forums and social media groups can offer invaluable information, solidarity and the opportunity to receive and give support. Participants share advice regarding fertility treatments and reviews of local doctors. They can support each other to get through difficult times and provide hope for the future. Many thousands of people set up special accounts for interacting with other infertility accounts, keeping it separate from their everyday social media interactions.

It is equally possible to have negative experiences, such as becoming emotionally affected by negative treatment results or miscarriages of online friends. Some also feel jealousy for those who have had successful treatments or given birth to a child. These are big emotions to feel for people you have never actually met in real life.

Be careful as the tips and advice offered online might not be scientifically evidence-based or appropriate for your situation. Though social media can make you feel a sense of connection, it still may not be a satisfactory substitute for real life support and social connection.

Even 'Fertility Influencers' and 'Fertility Coaches' can be detrimental to your resilience as you progress through infertility treatment. Some of them can be overly negative and depressing. Remember, you have the power to unfollow anyone who makes you feel defeated and doesn't help you stay focused, happy and healthy on your journey to achieve your fertility goals.

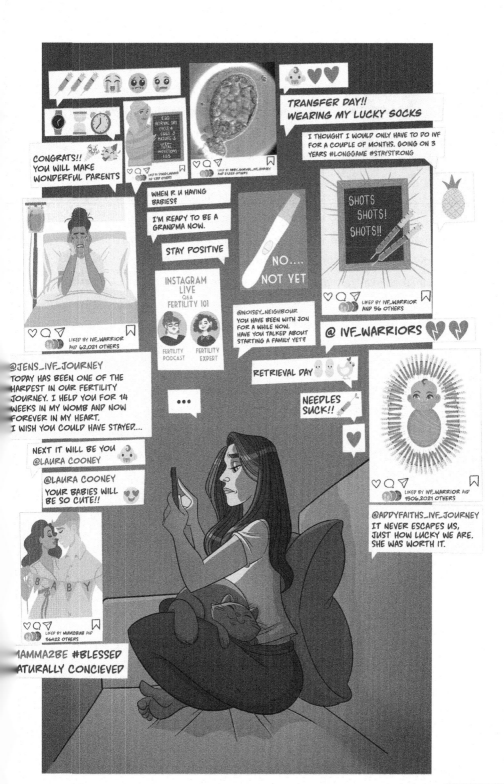

FROM LAURA

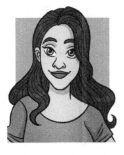

When we first started IVF, I wanted to understand what was about to happen to me. How would it feel physically? How would the experience impact me emotionally? No one in my life had been through fertility treatment, so there was no one I could ask. While doctors and nurses could explain the procedures, they couldn't really help me understand what it would feel like.

After looking around online, I stumbled on some channels where people shared raw and real videos of their fertility treatment. I could watch and empathise with their real-life experiences. This prepared me better than anything else.

Later, when we became more experienced with IVF, we shared our own story online, hoping to help others who are lost at the start, like I was.

Follow us on social media @InfertilityMan or go to www.InfertilityMan.com

▶ Pay attention to how you approach infertility online and make sure it is a positive experience.

▶ Take any fertility advice received online with a grain of salt. It may not be evidence-based and should not replace the advice of your doctor. If anyone online makes you feel bad, unfollow them.

▶ Be aware of how you and your partner are responding to social media. If it is affecting your mental health or taking up too much of your time, take a break.

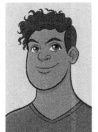

*My partner would say that joining the online communities was a turning point for her. At the start of our fertility treatment we were quite private, but then one day out of sheer frustration and desperation she just started looking around online and stumbled across these wonderful communities. It made a major difference. I believe it contributed significantly to the resilience that she showed, which until then she didn't even know that she had. It helped me too, because she had other outlets, she had other supports apart from me. - **Amir**

BABY-MAKING MEET UP

Being united with your baby-making team is so important as you interact with the rest of the world.

- ▶ Discuss any times when you have felt sad or uncomfortable around pregnant people, babies, or children. How can you manage these emotions? How can you support each other?

- ▶ Have a laugh about the ridiculous things people say about having or not having children. Try to find the funny side in their complete lack of empathy. Remind yourselves that even though these comments can hurt, you can choose to ignore them. And most of the time the intention is good, it is the execution that is flawed.

- ▶ Discuss any upcoming events that might be difficult while you are experiencing infertility. Work out a plan for how you can support each other.

- ▶ How will you navigate the online world while trying to conceive? Which social media accounts or groups make you feel empowered and which ones should you avoid? Who do you need to unfollow? How can you help each other interact with social media and the internet in a positive way?

- ▶ Join an infertility group online; we have one for men called The Men's Infertility Group, check www.InfertilityMan.com for details.

FERTILITY TREATMENT

FERTILITY VOCABULARY

Finally, we have reached the point where we will talk about medical treatments for infertility. Before we discuss the next steps, we need to learn a whole new language. Were you aware that infertile people have their own secret language?

Generally, women tend to be more fluent in 'Fertilese' and they speak it in the many online support groups for infertility. Doctors can also use it occasionally. Most of it is abbreviations. I guess when that biological clock is ticking, anything that saves a bit of time is a good thing.

Join an infertility group online; we have one for men called The Men's Infertility Group, check www.InfertilityMan.com for details.

In these groups, you will see sentences like this:

TTC for 2 years with a FS, diagnosed with Endo, low AMH and a poor SA – AF always arrives and it's a BFN. We are currently 5DP5DT, IVF with ICSI of one PGT embaby. If this doesn't work, we'll do an FET and after that, DH and I will be back to BD. But right now, we are PUPO! Hopefully PASP!

Can you decipher that?

It means …

Trying to conceive for 2 years with a fertility specialist, diagnosed with endometriosis, low anti-Müllerian hormone and a poor sperm assessment – Aunt Flo (meaning a woman's period) always arrives and it's a big fat negative (meaning a negative pregnancy test). We are currently 5 days past 5-day transfer (meaning 5 days have passed since transferring a 5-day-old embryo back into the woman's uterus), In vitro fertilisation with intracytoplasmic sperm injection (meaning the sperm was injected into the egg) of one pre-implantation genetically tested embryo. If this doesn't work, we'll do a frozen embryo transfer and after that, Dear Husband and I will be back to baby dancing (having sex, hoping to conceive). But right now, we are pregnant until proven otherwise! Hopefully pregnant and staying pregnant!

It's quite a mouthful!

You don't need to learn to speak this new language, but having a basic understanding (and the glossary at the end of this book) is just another way to support your partner and to understand what is happening.

So, if you hear a term or an abbreviation that you don't understand, either ask in the moment for it to be explained or look it up. Pretending to understand will get you nowhere, as will zoning out of the conversation. Once you can decipher the language, it can be quite fun. It's nice to have a secret language with the infertility club – a club that no one wants to join but a club that has incredible members.

FERTILITY TREATMENTS

When people think about fertility treatments, their minds immediately jump to IVF. However, there are other less expensive and less invasive options you can try before going with IVF. Low-tech treatments do not involve fertilisation outside of the uterus, so they are less complicated to perform. For many people, these treatments can be a way to supercharge their fertility and get them over the line to achieve a pregnancy. For others, these are a choice that should be bypassed, as they will find more success by focusing their time, money and energy on IVF. Your choice will depend on your diagnosis, your age and how you choose to allocate your resources.

Cycle Tracking

Ovulation cycle tracking is a simple process that can help a woman identify which days she's most fertile. The doctor will track her hormone cycle to predict when ovulation is going to take place with a high degree of accuracy.

Ovulation is triggered by a surge of hormones from the pituitary gland. By carrying out simple blood and ultrasound tests to detect this hormone surge, the doctor can advise you of the ideal time to have sex to give you the best chance of conception. Cycle tracking with a clinic is more accurate than ovulation prediction kits and temperature tracking at home.

Ovulation Induction

Ovulation induction (OI) is for women who may or may not ovulate regularly and who have normal fallopian tubes and male partners with regular sperm quality.

The treatment involves stimulating the woman's ovaries with medication and the follicular growth monitored with blood tests and ultrasound scans. When the size of the follicle and the oestrogen level suggests that the egg is soon to be released (ovulation) the patient is advised to have intercourse. It is a common first step along the fertility treatment journey.

It's important to use medications under the care of a fertility specialist, as the woman's cycle will be closely monitored to check the size and number of follicles present to avoid multiple pregnancies.

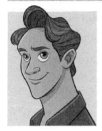 *I feel like this is not spoken about often enough, especially amongst men. But I do, I speak with my friends and my colleagues. I think everybody feels as though they are the only one going through this experience, that they can't talk to anyone about it, that they should hide it, you know all that nonsense that we self-inflict. I don't hide it because I feel it needs to be spoken about more. The taboo needs to be removed because going through fertility treatment is crushing even when you know what to expect. But when you don't know what to expect, it's even harder. - Xavier*

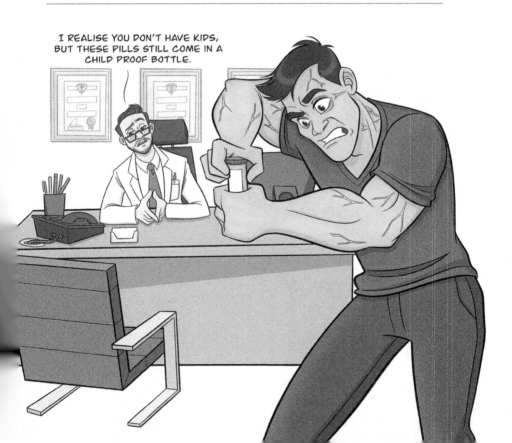

Flushing the Fallopian Tubes

This technique effectively clears a woman's fallopian tubes by flushing them with liquid to allow her eggs to travel unhindered into the uterus. It is generally carried out as part of an exploratory HSG or hysteroscopy. Obviously, this will improve things if blocked tubes are your only issue. Tubal flushing has several advantages over IVF, including that the benefit persists over time while IVF only helps for the one cycle. Tubal flushing helps achieve an otherwise natural conception and is much cheaper than other fertility treatments.

Intrauterine Insemination IUI

Sometimes called artificial insemination, alternative insemination, or donor insemination. Sperm that have been washed and concentrated are placed directly into the woman's uterus around the time her ovary releases an egg to be fertilised. This helps the best sperm to get closer to the egg. It is often combined with fertility drugs and blood tests to pinpoint ovulation timing. IUI has statistically lower chances of success than IVF, but it is much cheaper and less invasive. IUI is often used if you have been diagnosed with unexplained infertility, hostile cervical mucus, minor sperm abnormalities or other male disorders. It can be used when sperm have been frozen because of the sperm provider's absence or due to chemotherapy or radiotherapy or when using donated sperm.

IVF

You have chosen a doctor, done some initial testing and decided that In Vitro Fertilisation (IVF) is the next step for you.

It is worth mentioning that every clinic and every doctor has their own way of doing things. We'll give a general overview of a typical IVF cycle, so you have an idea of what is going to happen next. Your experience will be unique, but hopefully understanding the process will help you navigate each stage.

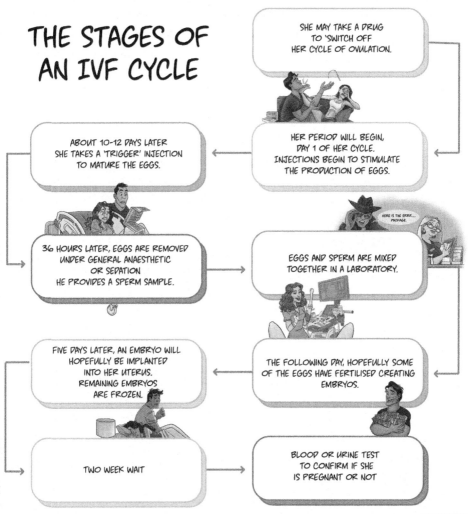

THE STAGES OF AN IVF CYCLE

SHE MAY TAKE A DRUG TO 'SWITCH OFF HER CYCLE OF OVULATION.

ABOUT 10-12 DAYS LATER SHE TAKES A 'TRIGGER' INJECTION TO MATURE THE EGGS.

HER PERIOD WILL BEGIN, DAY 1 OF HER CYCLE. INJECTIONS BEGIN TO STIMULATE THE PRODUCTION OF EGGS.

36 HOURS LATER, EGGS ARE REMOVED UNDER GENERAL ANAESTHETIC OR SEDATION HE PROVIDES A SPERM SAMPLE.

EGGS AND SPERM ARE MIXED TOGETHER IN A LABORATORY.

FIVE DAYS LATER, AN EMBRYO WILL HOPEFULLY BE IMPLANTED INTO HER UTERUS. REMAINING EMBRYOS ARE FROZEN.

THE FOLLOWING DAY, HOPEFULLY SOME OF THE EGGS HAVE FERTILISED CREATING EMBRYOS.

TWO WEEK WAIT

BLOOD OR URINE TEST TO CONFIRM IF SHE IS PREGNANT OR NOT

THE STAGES OF AN IVF CYCLE

The beginning of an IVF cycle can be met with mixed emotions: impatience to start the process, reluctance to begin injections, nerves, hope, excitement and even fear. And all these feelings will come at the same time. Be prepared for this range of emotions both in yourself and in your baby making team. Be gentle with yourself and each other as you process how you're feeling.

Regulate

First, your partner may or may not have to go on the contraceptive pill, depending on the type of protocol you and your doctor have selected. This is just to get her cycle regular and perhaps help to line it up with certain dates. Some clinics may have her do something called down regulation (sometimes known by its nickname downregging). This is essentially the process of shutting down her hormones to stop the natural process of ovulation by injecting or sniffing a medication. Some protocols do not include regulation, so you might skip this stage all together.

Stimulate

Your partner will pay attention to her cycle and wait for Day 1 of her period, which means the first day of 'full flow'. This means that her period has started and is properly flowing, not just 'spotting'.

As soon as her period begins in earnest, you will call the fertility clinic and let them know your cycle has begun. You will already have a fridge full of medications or you will run out and grab them that day. This stage involves injecting drugs that mirror her natural hormones and stimulate her ovaries to produce follicles and hopefully, lots of eggs.

Many women find this process difficult for two main reasons. First, it is not a lot of fun to inject yourself at regular times every day. Second, the drugs can have some uncomfortable side effects. Physically, she can have pain in her tummy as the drugs cause her ovaries to go into overdrive and she might have a very bloated midsection. She may just have general feelings of being unwell, such as headaches and nausea.

Additionally, she may experience heightened emotions. She might feel intensely aggravated, sad, angry or even out of control due to some raging hormones, similar to premenstrual tension (PMT). Alternatively, she may feel fine, each person responds to the medications differently.

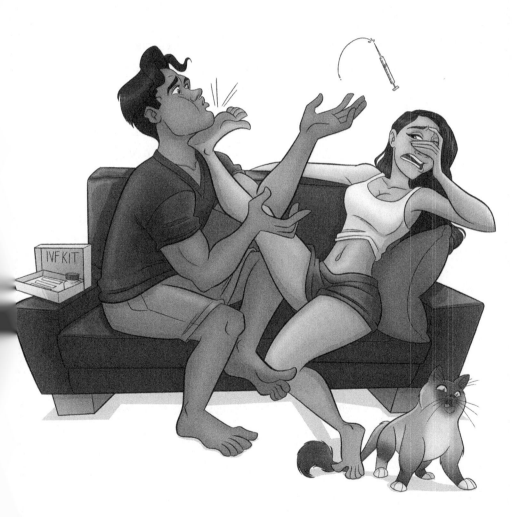

FROM LAURA

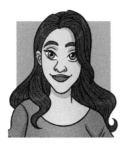

When Jon and I started out with IVF, I didn't want to do my own injections. I mean, who would? It made sense since he was a paramedic, that he would give me my injections. He was super supportive and we both went out of our way to make sure we were together, every day, twice a day when it was time to administer the shots.

As our IVF journey continued (much longer than we expected it would) it became impossible to continue on like that. Jon was working a lot on the ambulance (IVF ain't cheap!) and my work was regularly taking me overseas.

So, the time came for me to do the injections myself. I knew what I was going to feel when I shoved the needle in, but the idea of doing it to myself still freaked me out. I don't know if you have ever stabbed yourself with a needle before...it is difficult to do! Mentally, it is challenging to push a foreign object into your skin.

Jon stepped up to help me and offered his own tummy for me to practice on. Of course, we kept everything clean and sterile with no medication in the syringe. He let me practice by simply pushing the needle into his skin and removing it. That really helped. It meant that the first time I had to learn to push a needle into skin, it wasn't my own skin. It still took me a full ten minutes to do it, but it really helped me to be ready.

The next time I needed to administer some medication to myself, I was brave enough to do it (after another ten minutes of psyching myself up). It wasn't too long before I was an expert, injecting myself in cars, public bathrooms and even on planes.

HOW TO ADMINISTER AN INJECTION

1. Be Involved

The first step is to involve yourself. Just because you may not be having the injections doesn't mean you're not part of the process. You're a team, you're in this together and your support will make an enormous difference to your partner.

When your doctor has selected the medications, have a look at the treatment protocol. The doctor, nurses and the pharmacist should give you some instructions on how to mix the vials and prepare the syringes. Make sure you get them to teach you at your pace and repeat the demonstration until you feel confident.

Offer to go to the pharmacy to collect the medications. You should be given syringes, injecting pens and needles, as well as alcohol swabs and a sharps container to dispose of used items safely. You won't know yet how long this stage of the cycle will last, so pharmacies usually give you enough for about 12 days. You may need to return for more medications if the stimulation part of the cycle takes longer than expected.

2. Create a Plan

Talk to your partner and find out when she thinks her period will start. Mark that date on your calendar (but be prepared that it may change). When Day 1 comes around, she will call the fertility clinic to let them know your IVF cycle has begun. Then you can work out your plan for the injections based on your treatment protocol – some may be in the morning and some in the evening.

You can usually choose the exact time as long as it is the same time each day, so choose a time that will suit you both. Let her know you would like to be there, even if she prefers to give the injections herself. Set an alarm to go off 15 minutes before each one. You can be very supportive by helping her to remember the injections each day.

3. Calm Yourself

Your job is to make this as easy as possible for her, and that means being a calming influence. The first step in helping her to be calm is to be calm yourself. Take a few deep breaths; go to another room if you need to.

4. Get Ready to Inject

First, wash your hands. Keeping things clean and sterile is important. She may want to prepare the medications herself, or she may be happy to hand that job over to you. Clean and clear a space on a table. Read through the treatment plan and collect everything you will need: the medications, the needles, the sharps container and an ice pack from the freezer. Use the alcohol wipes provided, wipe every surface or vial that will get pricked when you are mixing the medications.

Check the paperwork, the dose and the timing. Check the paperwork again. Ask your partner to check the paperwork. Having two people check the details prevents mistakes.

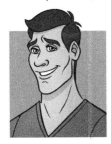

FROM JON: *I'm a paramedic and in that job we check the medications again and again to prevent mistakes. We read the dosage amounts out loud to each other and get our colleague to sign off. It's a good idea to do this during IVF too.*

Ask her to choose the spot where she would like to be injected, usually on her stomach. Avoid injecting on top of any bruises, which can hurt more. While it is not necessary, many people like to numb the area using an ice pack. Some people like to use a numbing cream or gel.

FROM JON: *Using ice for subcutaneous injections seemed unnecessary to me – we would never do that in the ambulance. However, it makes complete sense when you have to do two or more injections per day for the better part of a month. The ice packs worked to soothe some tender and bruised areas before*

having to inject again. The ice packs were also useful for keeping the medication at
the required temperature when we were injecting away from home.

Although skin that is visibly soiled or dirty must be washed, it may be
unnecessary to wear gloves and alcohol swab the skin before giving a
subcutaneous injection (an injection that goes into the fat, rather than a vein
or muscle). However, if you have alcohol wipes, there is no harm in doing it.
Use them to swab the area and allow to dry for 30 seconds before injecting.
You might even like to make her laugh by putting on your gloves and playing
up your role.

FROM JON: *Laura is very specific about where on her body she wants me to*
inject. I play a little joke by swabbing a place completely different to where
Laura has selected, and it always gets a laugh, which lightens the mood and
relieves some tension prior to injecting.

Tip: When you come together for the injections, take some time to connect.
Make a ritual out of it, have a chat about your day, talk briefly about how
you're feeling about the fertility treatment and if appropriate, give her a
kiss. The repetitive nature of these injections can be linked to some caring
and kind interactions so that you can look forward to these moments, rather
than dreading them.

FROM JON: *It was a good chance to talk about how we were both feeling*
and to remind ourselves of the outcome we were hoping for through IVF. We
kept these moments as positive as we possibly could.

However, don't sit around chatting for too long. Sometimes Laura would
try to stall the injection by talking. You need to take your injections at the
same time each day, so sometimes you might need to hurry things along and
encourage her to get it done.

5. Give the Injections

Get yourself into a good position where you can easily reach her, because it's time to inject! If you have to do more than one injection, it can work well to start with the injection that hurts the most (she will know which one she likes the least.) Best to get that one over with and then you have the easy ones left to do.

Pinch a good chunk of the skin and hold it firmly. Push the needle in with confidence. A timid approach may not pierce the skin which can hurt a lot, the needle needs a bit of pressure behind it. Kind of like popping a balloon – if you press too softly the skin won't break immediately, but if you give it a bit of momentum, you get that instant pop. It's kind of like a dart going into a dartboard, it needs a bit of force in order to penetrate. Once the needle has broken through the skin, slowly and gently inject all the fluid.

FROM JON: *After the initial jab, Laura likes me to stop pinching her skin and for the fluid to be injected very, very slowly. Almost glacially slow. Weirdly, once the needle is in, you can use your other hand to give her a gentle tickle somewhere else on her stomach. This distracts her mind from the site of the injection, confusing her senses and reducing the sting. Strange, but it seems to work. It might also make her smile.*

Once the fluid has all been pushed in, wait for a few seconds before removing the needle. This prevents the fluid from popping back out again, although if that happens, it's nothing to worry about. Pull the needle out gently, at the same angle that it went in. Sometimes it might bleed a little. Again, nothing to worry about, though very annoying if it gets on her clothes. Apply some pressure and the bleeding will stop.

Be cool if she gives you feedback on your technique – it's not personal. Having an injection everyday hurts and she might have some ideas on how to make it hurt less. It is best to listen and assure her you will do your best to take her feedback on board for next time.

Dispose of your used needles safely in a sharps container and put any medications back in the fridge. Clear everything away – you don't want to be looking at it all day long.

Tip: Some women like to keep their needles until the end of their fertility treatment so that they can look back on how many injections they were brave enough to do. Some even like to take a photo of them, so don't throw anything away without asking her and make sure that the needles are stored in a safe container.

6. Celebrate Together

Going through fertility treatment is challenging, so celebrate every small thing you can. Giving yourself or your partner an injection is an act of bravery. Celebrate by complimenting her on how awesome she is, give each other a high five, a cuddle or whatever is appropriate for your relationship.

Some days she may find injections challenging, some days they may be totally easy. As her support person, listen and respond to what she needs on that particular day.

FROM JON: *Once we finished each injection, I would give her a kiss and she would say "Is everything going to be ok?" and I would say, "Everything is already ok. I love you and thank you for everything you are doing."*

Tip: Before you put everything away, do a little stock take. Keep track of the medications you have and how many more days they will last. Make sure there is no need for any last-minute dashes to the pharmacy.

What if we miss an injection?

If you make a mistake with your injections, it's not necessarily the end of the world (or the cycle). The first step is to calm down and get in touch with your doctor or nurse as soon as you can. Many fertility clinics provide after-hours contact details for this situation. Your doctor will advise if the missed medication will have any impact on your cycle.

If you can't get in touch with them immediately, continue on with your protocol as accurately as possible, even if a dose is a couple of hours late. Do not inject two doses at the same time to make up for the missed dose.

FROM JON: *Once Laura was at home injecting by herself and she gave herself the evening meds instead of the morning meds – mistakes can happen. We got in touch with our doctor and she told us what to do. Everything worked out ok.*

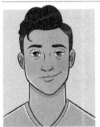

All the feelings, the guilt, the fear, we go through it too as the partner of someone doing fertility treatment. We think, 'I feel terrible, but I shouldn't be allowed to feel terrible because she is the one who has to go through all the injections and the procedures.' It is a complex set of emotions that men feel and we're not always great at dealing with that. Anything that can help men who need help – because lots of us do – I think it's fantastic. - Chris

ULTRASOUNDS AND BLOOD TESTS

While she is injecting to stimulate her ovaries to produce more eggs, she will need to have regular progress checks. Your doctor will keep track of how the follicles and potential eggs are developing and check the hormone levels with vaginal ultrasounds and blood tests.

Go with your partner to her first scan of the cycle if you can. Towards the end of the cycle, she may have to go in for scanning every second day, and it's understandable that you may not make it to every appointment. The first scan is important because that is when she will get her first 'report card'. This is the first time that she gets an idea of how many follicles are developing and therefore how many eggs she is likely to produce. It's great if you can be there because, depending on her expectations, she will want to celebrate with you if things are looking good, or she may need comforting if it's not going as well as expected.

The doctor will look at her scans and blood test results to make decisions about her ongoing treatment. They might decide to increase or decrease her medication, book her in for more ultrasounds, change the number of days that she needs to keep injecting or cancel the cycle.

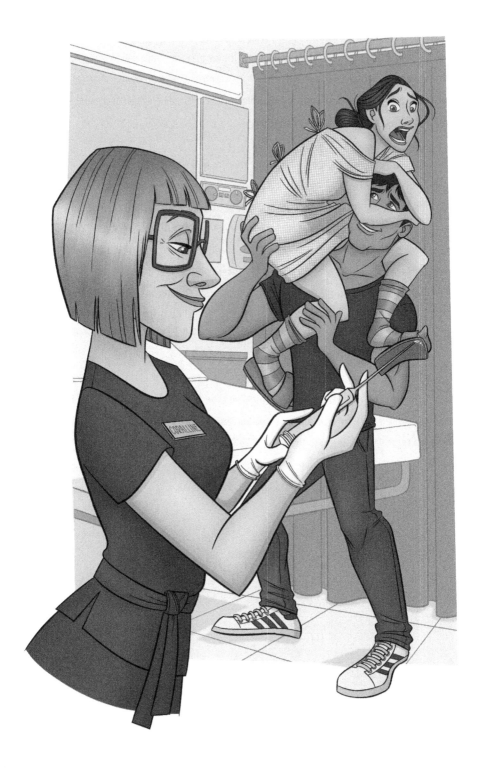

Trigger

When the follicles are looking good and a decent portion have reached the optimal size (usually as close as possible to 20 mm) then it's time to trigger. Getting to this stage takes a different amount of time for each woman, between 9 and 20 days.

Your fertility clinic will tell you an exact time to administer the trigger injection. It is important that you do it on time, as they set it up to match with the surgical schedule on the day of egg retrieval. This gives the eggs the optimal amount of time to be ready for retrieval, usually 36 hours. You might even need to get up during the night for the trigger shot. If you can, let her sleep. You can take responsibility for mixing the medication and making sure you get the timing right. Set two alarms to make sure you're on time.

Take a moment to celebrate getting to this stage. Do something nice for her, make a little speech thanking her for everything she has done so far, or clink a glass of tea together to celebrate.

Top Tip

Ask your doctor why they are choosing this timing for your trigger shot. The doctor will make careful decisions about the timing of your cycle and it can be useful for you to understand their thought process.

At your partner's ultrasound, it may be possible to see several follicles in her ovaries and they may be different sizes. The sonographer will measure the size of the follicles at each ultrasound. Generally, follicles grow about 2mm per day during an IVF cycle.

Typically, mature eggs may be found in follicles that measure between 12mm and 20mm at the time of egg retrieval. If the follicles are smaller or larger, then they are less likely to produce mature eggs. The doctor will decide on the timing of the egg collection, giving priority to the follicles that have responded best to the medications and are most likely to produce a mature egg.

By asking your doctor why they are making certain choices about your cycle, you can ensure that they are paying close attention and also learn for yourself about how her body is responding during IVF.

EGG AND SPERM RETRIEVAL

Eggs

Finally, it's the Big Day! Your partner will need to fast to prepare for her surgery, which means no food or drink. Be considerate of this and don't show off your breakfast to her. She might feel anxious, so do your best to calm her worries and don't take anything too personally.

At the hospital, the anaesthetist will put her to sleep and then the surgeon will place a device into the vagina that pushes a needle through the vaginal wall and into each ovary. Once the needle is inside, it is manoeuvred to pierce one follicle after another, guided by ultrasound. Suction pulls the fluid out through a tube and hopefully floating within the extracted fluid will be her eggs.

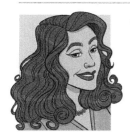

*Some patients worry that IVF will use up all their eggs, but that is not correct. Every month she has a pool of eggs and at the end of the month, those eggs have died. All your doctor is doing with IVF is 'egg rescuing' by retrieving those eggs that were going to die. It's an egg rescue mission. - **Dr Lynn Burmeister***

Sperm

While she is in surgery, you will give your sperm sample if you are able to retrieve sperm the usual way. Most clinics these days suggest you bring your own adult entertainment. Saliva, lubricants and creams should be avoided, as they can have an adverse effect on the sample. The beginning of the ejaculate is the most concentrated part of the sample, so aim to get it all in the cup. Avoid touching the inside of the cup and if any semen spills, do not attempt to transfer it to your cup. As soon as you've collected your sample, put the lid on your container. Make sure that the name and other details on the cup are correct.

Don't worry about the amount of fluid you collect. Remember that it is more about the quality of the sperm than the quantity of the seminal fluid. If you are producing your sample at home, carry it in your pocket as you take it to the clinic, to keep it at body temperature.

Recovery

Once you have provided your sample, it will be time to collect your partner from her surgery. The egg retrieval surgery itself is quite quick, usually between 15 and 30 minutes. Your partner will take some time to wake up from the anaesthesia. Make sure your phone is nearby, as the nurses will call you to collect her.

An egg retrieval is considered minor surgery and your partner will most likely be able to come home within a few hours. Nonetheless, it is still a surgical procedure that carries potential risks and can be uncomfortable. As soon as she is discharged, take her home to bed with a heat pack on her tummy and painkillers as directed. After fasting and the general anaesthetic she may be quite hungry and thirsty, so organise her favourite meal and keep her fluids up. She should be feeling better in a few days, hopefully she can take some time off to relax at home.

EXPECTATION VERSUS REALITY

Egg Numbers

From her ultrasounds during the stimulation phase, you will have an idea of how many follicles are present, which will give you an idea of how many eggs you can expect to retrieve.

When your partner wakes up from surgery, her doctor will tell her how many eggs they were able to retrieve. Sometimes they will tell her in person and sometimes they will write a number on her hand or a piece of paper for her to see post surgery (when she is still groggy from the general anaesthetic).

If she expects to collect lots of eggs and she only gets a few, she might be very disappointed. An IVF cycle is a lot to go through, to then retrieve what she thinks is a small number of eggs, or in some cases, no eggs at all. Let her know she can call you as soon as the nurses bring her phone to her and that you will be waiting to hear from her.

Sometimes women can hear the results of other women on the ward and compare themselves. Dashed hopes and comparison could make you and her feel pretty dejected after all your hard work.

Only some of the eggs retrieved will be mature. An egg is mature after it has undergone two separate rounds of meiosis or cell division. These rounds of cell division reduce the number of chromosomes in the nucleus of the egg from 46 to 23. At some point during the day when your partner is recovering at home, she will get a phone call from the fertility clinic to let her know how many eggs have been identified as mature in the lab. Only mature eggs can be fertilised or frozen, the rest will be discarded. It can be upsetting to hear that the number of eggs has reduced.

Be supportive of your partner and let her express her disappointment. Give her a hug and let her know you are disappointed too. Depending on your situation, perhaps remind her you only need a few good quality eggs to be successful.

IVF involves trial and error. The doctor needs to get a sense of how she responds to the medications. If you are disappointed with your numbers, plan a follow-up appointment with your doctor to ask if there is a way to make the next IVF cycle more successful. The doctor should be able to alter the dosages and types of medications to find the mix that works best for your partner.

Ovarian Hyperstimulation Syndrome (OHSS)

Occasionally, women may suffer from ovarian hyperstimulation syndrome during or after their IVF cycle. This is a very serious condition that can cause blood clots, kidney failure or even death (in extremely rare cases). This is one reason why women are monitored so closely during IVF. If your partner starts experiencing symptoms like abdominal pain, nausea and vomiting during her IVF cycle, get in touch with your fertility clinic as soon as possible.

She may be hesitant to report it because she is worried about her IVF cycle being cancelled, but your job first and foremost, is to keep her safe. In many cases, the IVF cycle will still go ahead and her eggs will be retrieved – and if it doesn't, it is still better to be safe than sorry.

If she has OHSS, the doctor may recommend freezing all the embryos and waiting a month. This gives her body some time to recover before the embryo is transferred back into her uterus with her next cycle. She may well be disappointed at the delay, but you can reassure her that this is the safest strategy to give that little embryo the best chance. Waiting to allow her body to be in the best shape to potentially begin a pregnancy is smart and it will mean that you aren't just wasting an embryo that her body is not ready to receive.

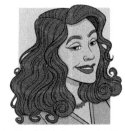 *OHSS is where the woman has an unusual reaction to the fertility medications. It is often caused by the trigger injection, which causes the eggs to ovulate and the ovaries to produce a hormone called VEGF, which dilates all her blood vessels and makes them leaky. So instead of the fluid staying in the blood vessels, it can leak into the abdomen or lungs, which can feel like drowning. Fortunately, the incidence of OHSS is low because if we suspect she might be getting close, we don't give the hCG trigger injection. We're very careful about that because we don't want our patients sitting in a hospital recovering from OHSS. It can be life threatening, it can be a very serious complication. Sometimes, even though we're being as careful as possible... we still see it.* **- Dr Lynn Burmeister**

What if the Cycle is Cancelled?

It can be very upsetting to have an IVF cycle cancelled before egg retrieval. Imagine injecting yourself for days and then being told that it's not working and you need to stop. Sometimes stopping means it's just not working this time and you can try again in a later month. Occasionally, it means that IVF will not work for you at all and the doctor will start talking to you about other options.

The first cycle may be cancelled because the doctor can see that they might get a better result if they try again with a better understanding of how she responds to the medications. The upside is that she doesn't have to go through an egg retrieval surgery, which would most likely give a poor result. Cancelling should also mean that you don't pay for a full cycle and you can save for the next attempt when you can be hopeful of a better outcome.

It is very challenging if the cycle was cancelled because the doctor doesn't believe that IVF with her own eggs is a viable option for you. This will be very hard to hear and you will need to support each other emotionally. Your doctor should arrange a follow-up appointment to discuss what happened during the cycle and what your options may be for the future. It is common for couples to experience grief when receiving this news. Work with your partner to help her make a list of questions that you would like to ask your doctor. Get the answers you need and hopefully some closure that helps you move to the next stage.

TREATMENTS FOR MALE FACTOR INFERTILITY

Infertility is sometimes caused by problems with the sperm, otherwise known as Male Factor Infertility. If that is your diagnosis, then this chapter is for you. If not, you may choose to skip ahead. Being informed about potential solutions for Male Factor Infertility can help when engaging with your medical professionals and deciding your course of action.

Vasectomy Reversals

Men who thought they were choosing to have no more children and underwent a vasectomy occasionally decide to have a reversal because of a change of circumstance or a change of mind. While it is possible for men who have had a vasectomy to retrieve sperm surgically and use IVF to fertilise eggs, a vasectomy reversal is generally recommended as a first step. It usually only requires a single procedure and has a high success rate for achieving the presence of sperm in the ejaculate.

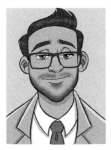

A Vasectomy Reversal is a highly technical procedure using sutures that are much thinner than human hair and the surgery takes up to 4-5 hours. The success rate depends on how you define success. If success is simply that the sperm comes back into the semen, if the procedure is done less than 7 years after the vasectomy, there is an 80-90% chance of success. That doesn't necessarily mean that the patient will have a child, as it takes two to tango and there are so many factors that come into achieving pregnancy. But at least if a patient has a successful vasectomy reversal, each month this couple is "at the starting gate" to try and conceive.
- Dr Darren Katz

Sperm Retrieval Procedures

If your sperm test comes back showing problems with volume, motility or morphology, you may still be able to have a biological child with medical assistance. Find a great doctor with expertise in male factor infertility to figure out the best strategy for you.

Even if you have very few sperm in your ejaculate, it may be possible to surgically retrieve it from within the testicle. IVF with intracytoplasmic sperm injection (ICSI) means that even with a small number of sperm, it may still be possible to fertilise eggs, make embryos and hopefully start a pregnancy.

FROM JON

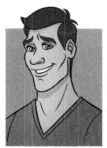

At first, I thought I couldn't have my own kids because my sperm count was a big fat zero. I had been diagnosed with Non-Obstructive Azoospermia, meaning I just didn't make a lot of sperm or maybe I didn't make any at all. When we looked a little deeper with the fine needle aspiration procedure, we found one immotile sperm. That one sperm gave us hope we might find more.

As we learned more about the various sperm retrieval surgical options, we decided not to do any biopsy procedures, as we didn't want to risk creating scar tissue within my one testicle. Instead, we jumped ahead to try the microTESE procedure. We were lucky enough to do it twice (which is unusual) and we found about 30 motile sperm each time.

Which sperm retrieval procedure is recommended?

When it comes to retrieving sperm there are various options available to you. Seek advice from a qualified urologist or fertility specialist who can help with your particular diagnosis.

Some doctors may recommend a certain procedure because they are not trained in the more complex forms of sperm extraction, such as the microTESE. Ask your doctor why they are recommending one procedure over another and if they are qualified in microsurgical sperm extraction. If you feel that your diagnosis may benefit from a more precise surgical procedure than your doctor is able to offer, seek a second opinion.

To keep it really simple, there are three main categories of sperm collection procedures.

► Sperm is aspirated with a needle
► Sperm is extracted through an incision, known as a biopsy
► Sperm is targeted using a surgical microscope and then extracted

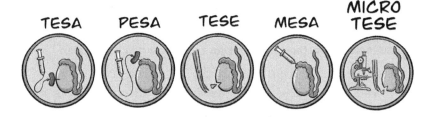

TESA   PESA   TESE   MESA   MICRO TESE

Needle Procedures

FNA – fine needle aspiration, TEFNA – testicular fine needle aspiration,

TESA Testicular Sperm Aspiration or PESA – percutaneous epididymal sperm aspiration

These procedures involve the insertion of a needle into the testicles under local anaesthetic. The doctor will insert the needle into the testicle, pull back on the syringe and hopefully find some sperm in the fluid. The procedure can be repeated until sufficient sperm is obtained. These are known as blind procedures, meaning the doctor cannot see where they are putting the needle. These quick and cost-effective procedures can be done in less than 20 minutes. However, as they are blind procedures, a problem is that they can cause some bleeding and scarring within the testicle that is hidden from the doctor because the procedures are done without visibility through the skin. Whilst in some men an FNA can be useful, a discussion needs to be had about whether a microTESE would be better first up (instead of FNA).

Testicular Biopsies

TESE –testicular sperm extraction
These procedures involve making a small incision in the testicles to remove tissue for further examination in the lab. This is called a biopsy and can be done under local or general anaesthetic.

As with needle procedures, biopsies can cause damage to the very sensitive tissue. Areas of bleeding can cause scar tissue within the testicle. If sperm is not found and a microTESE needs to be done later on, the scarring can make it much harder for the micro-surgeon to find the 'needle in a haystack', in other words, sperm.

Microscopic Testicular Biopsies

These procedures require general anaesthesia and a highly skilled micro-surgeon.

MESA – microsurgical epididymal sperm aspiration
MESA uses a surgical microscope to help retrieve sperm from the epididymis tubes.

MicroTESE – microsurgical testicular sperm extraction
During the microTESE procedure under general anaesthetic, the doctor uses a surgical microscope to examine the tubules at the time of the surgery. It's more accurate than a biopsy, as the doctor can see possible pockets of sperm up very close. They then selectively remove 'better' or more normal appearing tubules. Once removed, the tubules are opened and examined under a very strong microscope. This process can take up to five hours and most often the patient is able to return home on the same day.

Urologist and Microsurgeon Dr Darren Katz explains the microTESE procedure:

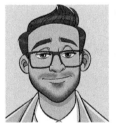

*Sperm only makes up around 1 or 2% of volume of the semen. That is why men with very little or no sperm often don't notice a difference in the volume of the semen. A lot of sperm must be made in the testicle in order to get a small amount to come out in the ejaculate. - **Dr Darren Katz***

In men who don't have any sperm in their ejaculate, we know that sometimes, somewhere within the testicle, there may be a tiny pocket where sperm is, in fact, being produced. Finding it is like finding a needle in a haystack. During the microTESE procedure, the surgeon looks thoroughly inside the testicle with a very high powered operating microscope hoping to find that one small area that looks like it might still be making sperm. The surgeon will then remove that tiny little piece, less than a millimetre. Inside the operating theatre there will be an embryologist present, who will look under an even higher-powered microscope, 400x power, and they're looking to see if that little piece of the testicle has sperm. During a microTESE, the surgeon will go through all parts of the testicle and get live, in-the-moment feedback from the embryologist.

If the team happens to get lucky and hit the jackpot early, then they will stop. However, if they don't find any in the first testicle, they will move to the other one. The operation can take several hours, it is quite labour intensive, though the patient will usually be able to return home on the same day. A doctor will normally only do one of these procedures a day because they need to really concentrate. In most men, you really just have one shot to do the microTESE, so you really want to make the first shot the best one. A man having more than one microTESE is the exception, not the rule. It is only possible if sperm is found very early in the first surgery, so the surgeon doesn't need to dissect the whole testicle. Usually there are not that many places in the testicle with sperm, sometimes there is only one. I remember one time with a patient several years ago, we were into the third hour before I found any sperm for this man.

It is a huge journey that patients have gone through before the man ends up on my operating table, usually years in the making. First, it's the time of trying to conceive naturally and then it's all the egg retrievals, all the hormonal changes, the prescriptions. For both of you, it's an emotional, physical, financial journey, and it all comes down to the microTESE. I know how much my patients have invested in this process, so it is up to me to invest as much as I can to give them the best possible outcome. So, I don't stop until I am confident that I have looked everywhere. - **Dr Darren Katz**

The challenge going in to sperm retrieval surgery is that it is very difficult to predict the likelihood of success in advance. It takes a lot of faith to sign yourself up for this surgery, knowing there is a chance that no sperm will be found or that the subsequent IVF process may be unsuccessful.

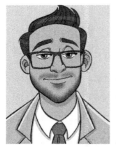 *There are only one or two genetic conditions where there is a zero percent chance of finding sperm and they are rare. Unfortunately, one or two times a year I have to tell patients that there is no point in doing a microTESE but for the vast majority of men who come into my clinic there is no test and no other findings that would preclude them from a microTESE.*

Of course, some have slightly more chance of being successful and some have slightly less, but there is no test that you can do beforehand that will tell you in advance whether your surgery will successfully find sperm. Most of the time, it would be very difficult to predict a patient's likelihood of success in advance.

This is why I don't recommend a 'diagnostic biopsy' in the majority of cases to work out what is going on, as it will not change my management, especially in patients who are not producing sperm. These patients need a microTESE as their first (and only) operation. The danger in doing a diagnostic biopsy is that it can cause scar tissue, making a microTESE more difficult. Also, if no sperm is found, then patients may need to wait up to 6 months before the microTESE can be performed to allow for healing to occur. Waiting for 6 months can potentially be problematic, especially if the female partner is of advanced maternal age. Waiting can be emotionally distressing.

Also, generally, a diagnostic biopsy is sent to a pathology laboratory to work out the cause of the problem. A diagnostic biopsy is random and what happens if, by chance, the doctor gets the only sperm available? That sperm then ends up at the pathology lab, rather than in the partner's egg!

- Dr Darren Katz

Questions to Ask Your Doctor:

▶ Are you convinced this is a production problem and not a blockage problem?

▶ Which procedure do you think would be give me the best chance of finding sperm in my case?

▶ Is there any procedure that you do not specialise in that might be more effective? Would it help to get a second opinion?

▶ How should I prepare for my procedure?

▶ Do you keep a personal record of your success rate for this particular treatment? If so, what is it?

How To Prepare for Your Sperm Retrieval

Preparing in the months leading up to your procedure may improve your chances of finding sperm. Eating healthy, avoiding excess coffee, getting plenty of sleep and potentially taking hormones prescribed by your doctor may improve the environment inside your body where sperm is produced.

THE THREE POTENTIAL PITFALLS OF MALE FACTOR INFERTILITY FROM JON

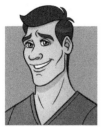

Male Factor Infertility is not often a topic of conversation. It is very difficult for men to find quality information to help them when they are faced with this diagnosis. Even the information that men receive from their doctors might not give them all that they need to make the right choices.

As we tried to seek treatment for my azoospermia, we discovered three potential pitfalls where men often make incorrect assumptions and decisions as they seek treatment. I certainly made mistakes with two of them and I almost did with the third. I believe that if I hadn't learned this information before making choices about my treatment, then it would have been unsuccessful. I shake my head in disbelief when I think about how close I came to almost ruining my chance of successfully retrieving sperm.

1. Supplementing Testosterone

Men with low testosterone may mistakenly assume that supplementing testosterone will help with their sperm production. Even doctors may prescribe it, not understanding the potential negative effect on male fertility.

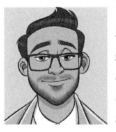

*There are two functions for the testicle: one is to make sperm and one is to make testosterone. And they often go hand in hand, but not always. This is because the sperm making parts of the testicle and the testosterone making parts of the testicle are separate. Often when somebody has severe problems with sperm production they also may have problems with testosterone levels. People try to do the right thing, they think 'I had better try to boost my testosterone', and they supplement with a testosterone medication they may have been prescribed or sourced themselves. That is, in fact, the worst thing they can do for their sperm - taking testosterone actually kills sperm. - **Dr Daren Katz**

---

2. Creating Scar Tissue in the Testicles

Every time you have a procedure on your testicles, you are creating scar tissue. If you pierce the testicle with a needle or operate on it in a biopsy procedure, the tissue inside will be damaged. Therefore it is very important to consider carefully which sperm retrieval procedure you choose.

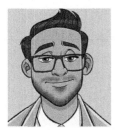 *When you operate on a testicle, it's a very fragile organ, it scars very easily. Even very limited biopsies can cause scar tissue. During a microTESE the surgeon is trying to find that 'needle in a haystack' so when there is scarring from previous biopsies instead of nice soft tissue, it is like trying to find a needle amongst concrete. I tell all my patients, your first shot at a sperm retrieval surgery should be your best shot. The vast majority of the patients who come to me who are not producing sperm will have a microTESE, not a little biopsy or fine needle aspiration or anything else. I don't think needle aspirations are that worthwhile, they are blind passes of a long, sharp needle into the testicle (meaning that the doctor cannot see where they are passing the needle). The needle is sort of just poked around. That can cause damage and make a future microTESE more difficult. Sometimes patients have a 'random biopsy' and they will take a piece of the testicle out in an operating theatre but without the microscope. These procedures can also cause lots of damage and scar tissue on occasions. Whilst there may be a role in certain circumstances for a limited 'random' biopsy, this is uncommonly needed and should be performed with a specialist who is experienced. It is mainly offered to where it is unclear if there is a sperm-making problem or if the ducts that carry the sperm are blocked. But usually, from blood tests, examination of the testicles by your specialist and some specialised imaging tests (e.g. ultrasound, MRI) the reason for no sperm is pretty obvious and a "diagnostic" biopsy is not needed. That is an important point, you don't want your doctor to decide, 'Well we'll just do a little fine needle aspiration, we'll do a little biopsy and we'll see what's in there.' You don't want that because what happens if they hit the lucky spot and find sperm, but they have damaged the only area that does produce sperm? That is a problem for when you want to do the microTESE later. - **Dr Darren Katz**

3. Not Having Enough Eggs

Eggs and sperm are single cells, which means they are less stable than embryos (which have multiple cells) when freezing and thawing. If you have male factor infertility, it is likely that sperm are difficult to find and potentially lower quality. Therefore, it is important to protect them as they undergo the necessary freezing and thawing as part of the IVF process. The safest place for sperm to be is inside eggs that have turned into embryos.

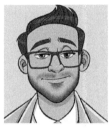

*In my practice, I use fresh sperm routinely because the partner's eggs are collected well in advance and they are kept in the freezer. The man undergoes the microTESE, if we find sperm, then the eggs are defrosted and injected, any excess sperm is frozen. I almost always use frozen eggs and fresh sperm. In my practice, I don't really use frozen sperm (unless there was excess left over from the microTESE). I am the first doctor in Australia to publish in a peer-reviewed journal a large series of microTESE operations using fresh sperm and the results are world class. In order to give fragile sperm the best shot, it is recommended to have a number of eggs ready before having a sperm retrieval procedure. The more eggs collected, the better, but it is always a balance of time, cost, side effects and the emotional and hormonal toll that egg collections can have. I generally prefer at least 10 frozen eggs prior to a microTESE. But if there are more, great. - **Dr Darren Katz**

FROM JON

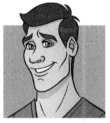

When anyone asks us about this, we always suggest doing at least one egg retrieval before you do the sperm retrieval, just to make sure that you have some eggs 'on ice'. Our doctor told us to have at least 20 of Laura's eggs already in the freezer so that they would be ready to be fertilised with any sperm they were able to find, so they would not need to be frozen on their own. We were also lucky enough to retrieve fresh eggs on the same day that we retrieved fresh sperm, but the frozen eggs gave us great peace of mind that my sperm would be made into embryos before going into the freezer.

Having Surgery to Find Sperm

FROM JON

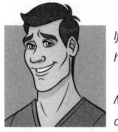

If it wasn't for the microTESE procedure, I would never have been able to have my own biological kids.

My first microTESE was meant to be my one and only chance. That is how we prepared for it anyway. Laura was doing egg retrievals to freeze enough eggs in advance (our doctor recommended at least 20) just in case I could produce the goods.

We planned for my procedure to take place on the same day as an egg collection for Laura so we would have fresh sperm (if they found any), and fresh eggs as well as the eggs that were already frozen. We ended up with 31 eggs in total.

It was an emotional day as I was about to find out once and for all whether there were any sperm hiding out in my testicles. It was a huge day for me, one I will never forget. Laura dropped me off at the hospital and I wandered in tentatively. I felt excitement, apprehension and fear but also a quiet optimism.

I put on my surgical gown and was wheeled into the operating room. The anaesthetist said to count down from 10, 9, 8, 7... and I was out for the count.

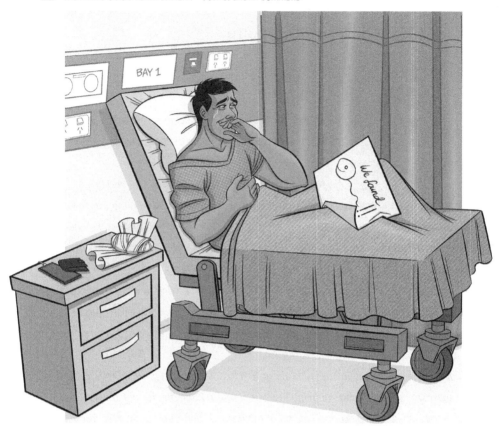

When I woke up groggy in the recovery ward, I found a piece of paper with
a hand drawn sperm and the words 'We found sperm'. Words cannot describe
how I felt in that moment. I'm not ashamed to say that I burst into tears.

As it happens, the doctor had found enough sperm early in the procedure and
made the call to close me back up. This meant I was going to be able to have
another bite at the cherry, if we chose to, I would be able to do the microTESE
a second time. Unbelievable!

See this moment on video at www.InfertilityMan.com/MansGuide

Recovery

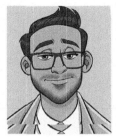

The microTESE is a very well tolerated procedure. Some men only require minimal pain relief medication, a bit of ice, supportive underwear and a few days of rest. Recovery can be uncomfortable, but not debilitating. Other patients may have different pain thresholds and be more sensitive down there. Some men may require consistent pain relief while they are recovering, for even up to a week. Everyone is different. **- Dr Darren Katz**

▶ Ice, ice and more ice. Soft gel ice packs are gentle and mould to the shape of your balls. Frozen vegetables also work well.

▶ Wear supportive underwear, but nothing too tight or restrictive.

▶ Your doctor may prescribe painkillers or recommend over-the-counter pain relief options.

▶ The drugs in your general anaesthesia and painkillers may cause constipation so have a plan to get things moving again.

▶ Drink lots of water and eat healthy food to help your digestive system get back on track.

▶ Take a break from exercise; your body needs a chance to recover.

▶ Rest. Take some time off work and get some good sleep if you can.

▶ Use your recovery time to feel proud of yourself for going through with your sperm retrieval. Whatever the outcome of your procedure, it's a brave thing to do. Whether you are happy or disappointed with the result, you can now move forward knowing you gave it your best shot.

Potential Long-Term Effects
of Sperm Retrieval Surgery

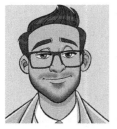

Probably the biggest and most common side effect that I get concerned about is permanently lowering a man's testosterone. Quite a lot of my patients already have lowered testosterone, so I know afterwards they are going to need testosterone anyway. There are also cases when before the sperm retrieval surgery, the man has normal testosterone, but about 10 – 15% of the time they end up needing long term, forever, testosterone replacement. That means obviously that the majority of men don't, but it is still a real risk for all of my patients.

Testosterone replacement is usually pretty straightforward, but it is something that patients need to be aware of before the surgery that it may be needed afterwards. Sometimes not right away, it could be years down the track. Most of the other risks are very rare. I'm dealing generally with otherwise healthy, fit, young men so the risks are pretty small.

- Dr Darren Katz

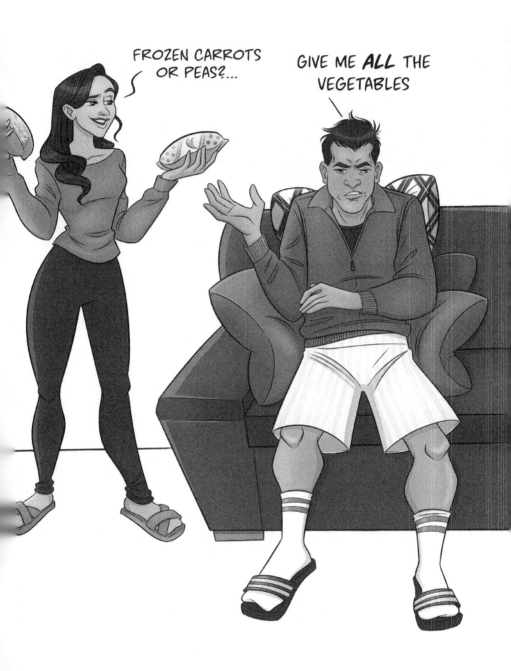

The Final Outcome

The microTESE success rate is varied. In my published data, the success rate for finding sperm in patients who are azoospermic is 61% for all patients. Because the success rate is varied from man to man, I generally say that in 50-60% of men I can find sperm. That means that around 40-50% of the men having this operation don't get the outcome that they want. So, you would think that half of the men would regret having had the operation and wish they had never done it. I can tell you I don't recall any man ever coming back and saying to me. 'Doc, why did I do this? This was the worst thing I have ever done.' That just never happens.

*Infertility is a psychological battle. For anyone who ends up on my operating table, it has been years in the making. It has been a long, long process. What the microTESE surgery does, is it allows them to close the book on that chapter in their life. They know that they have had the best available treatment in the world and whatever the outcome is; they know it is the final outcome for them. So, if they find sperm, brilliant! If they don't find sperm, they can put their head on the pillow at night and know that they have done everything they could, there are no regrets. The microTESE procedure gives people closure and they can just move on to whatever the next step is in their fertility journey. - **Dr Darren Katz***

FERTILISATION AND TESTING

On the day of the collection, it's time for the eggs to meet the sperm. Embryologists will 'wash' the sperm before introducing it to the eggs. Individual sperm are separated from the semen, removing any mucus and non-motile sperm to improve the chances of fertilisation.

To put it simply, there are two ways for the sperm to meet the eggs. The first way is plain old IVF, when thousands of sperm are placed in a petri dish with the egg and left to do their thing. Hopefully, one sperm will make its way inside the egg, just as it would if it were inside the body.

Alternatively, you may do an ICSI cycle, otherwise known as an intracytoplasmic sperm injection. The sperm get a little more help from the embryologist who will choose a single sperm and inject it into the egg. ICSI is used when there are a small number of sperm or when the sperm aren't in good enough shape to fight it out and swim to the egg.

The day after your egg and sperm retrievals, the clinic will call to let you know how many have fertilised and become embryos. The number of eggs that will fertilise depends on a variety of factors relating to egg and sperm quality and honestly, it is difficult to know why some eggs fertilise and some don't. On average, the number will drop by about 50% at this stage.

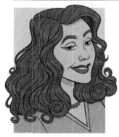

There is often a big drop off in numbers, it depends on the egg and sperm quality. We usually say that out of four eggs that get fertilised, you could expect that one of them will become a blastocyst. Be prepared for a major drop down. **- Dr Lynn Burmeister**

Incubation

Once the sperm are inside the eggs, it is a case of waiting to see what happens. Hopefully, they will develop into embryos and eventually a baby. Unfortunately, not all of them do. Over the next five days, you will get calls from your embryologist letting you know how your embryos are doing. Your number will probably drop again at this stage and some embryos will stop growing. On average, you can expect your number to go down by another 50%. Most clinics will transfer an embryo into the uterus or freeze them on Day 5 (and sometimes Day 6 or 7) when some embryos have hopefully reached blastocyst stage.

DAY 0	EGG RETRIEVAL AND INSEMINATION	
DAY 1	FERTILISATION	
DAY 2	CLEAVAGE STAGE (4 CELLS)	
DAY 3	CLEAVAGE STAGE (8 CELLS)	
DAY 4	MORULA STAGE	
DAY 5+	BLASTOCYST STAGE	
	BLASTOCYST STAGE/ HATCHING STAGE	

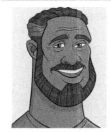

I still remember our first cycle. We had eleven embryos and seven of them fertilised. We got to Day 3, and all seven were still going really strong, the embryologist said they were all looking pretty good. And then on Day 4, we went from seven to one... and then nothing. - **Michael**

EMBRYO GRADING

Even after coming all this way, your remaining embryos still have some hurdles to jump. The embryologist will observe them and give them a grade. Embryo grading is sometimes called a 'beauty contest' because the embryologist can only go by what they can see. Sometimes great-looking embryos don't result in pregnancies and sometimes really ugly embryos do. Grading gives some indication of the likelihood of success and helps choose which embryo should be transferred first.

PRE-IMPLANTATION GENETIC TESTING

Pre-implantation genetic testing (PGT), also known as pre-implantation genetic screening (PGS), pre-implantation genetic diagnosis (PGD), or pre-implantation genetic testing for aneuploidies (PGT-A) is additional testing that looks at the chromosomal makeup of the embryos that make it to blastocyst stage. In simple terms, when the sperm and the egg come together, they each bring half a set of chromosomes with them, making a full set of 23 pairs (or 46 chromosomes). Sometimes there is a chromosome missing or there is an extra chromosome which can cause conditions such as Down syndrome, Trisomy 18, Trisomy 16 or Klinefelter syndrome. Chromosomal abnormalities can also cause miscarriage and other problems in pregnancy.

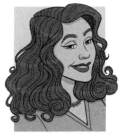

Pre-implantation genetic testing is not 100% accurate, but it is very close. Pregnancy rates from tested embryos are higher than from untested embryos. The science is there that it does work. For example, if you're 37 years old and you transfer a tested embryo, you chance of getting pregnant is 55% with a 15% miscarriage rate, whereas if you use an untested embryo you have a 35% chance of pregnancy and a 33% chance of miscarriage. Testing your embryo will increase your chance of having a live birth and decrease your chance of miscarriage. It's important to understand that PGS can only test the embryos you have to help find the right embryo sooner, it cannot increase your number of 'good' embryos. It helps you avoid going through transfer after transfer with embryos that wouldn't have made it. - Dr Lynn Burmeister

PGS or PGT testing is an optional extra and incurs additional costs. Only embryos that have reached blastocyst stage can be tested. The embryologist will need to freeze all your embryos if you want to wait for the results before transferring, which can take a couple of weeks. You should be aware that the results of these tests are not 100 percent accurate and the results still do not guarantee a successful transfer. Ask your doctor for additional information to decide if testing is a good idea for you.

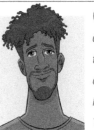

We had one AA graded embryo, it looked as perfect as you are going to get. We sent it off for PGD testing thinking, 'This is it, this is the super embryo, this is the one that is going to get us our baby.' It came back as PGD abnormal.

The funny story for us is that our son did not come from our best-looking embryo. The test result for his embryo came back inconclusive, one in three hundred chance and insufficient genetic material to do the test. As it turns out, he was the one! - Lamar

ADD ON TREATMENTS

Let's take a moment to talk about 'add ons'. These are optional additional treatments that your fertility clinic may provide, usually at extra cost. Here are some procedures that might be considered 'add on'.

▶ **Artificial Egg Activation**
When the sperm meets the egg, it triggers a process called 'egg activation'. Chemicals added to the liquid that the egg is placed into in the lab can stimulate this process.

▶ **Assisted Hatching**
Before an embryo can implant in the womb, it has to break out or 'hatch' from its zona pellucida. The embryologist can use lasers or other tools to make a hole, assisting it to 'hatch'

▶ **Endometrial Receptivity Array (ERA)**
This test claims to find the optimal time for embryo transfer by taking a biopsy of the endometrial lining. In following months, this information can be used to estimate the best possible time in the patient's cycle to transfer an embryo.

▶ **Endometrial Scratching**
During this procedure, the lining of the womb is 'scratched'. In theory, the procedure triggers the body to repair the site of the scratch, releasing hormones and chemicals that make the womb lining more receptive to an embryo implanting.

▶ **Embryo Glue (Hyaluronate enriched medium)**
Hyaluronate enriched medium is added to the dish in which the embryos are kept at the time of transfer, which may improve the chance of the embryo implanting.

► **Immunological tests and treatments**

In some patients, it is believed that their immune system could 'reject' the embryo as a foreign object within the body. These treatments can alter and suppress the immune system during early pregnancy.

► **Intracytoplasmic morphological sperm injection (IMSI)**

This technique involves using a microscope to view sperm under very high magnification (over x6000) hoping to identify the best sperm for fertilisation.

► **Physiological intracytoplasmic sperm injection**

This is used to select sperm by placing them in hyaluronic acid (HA) and identifying sperm that can bind to HA. These sperm are selected for use in treatment.

► **Pre-implantation genetic testing**

Embryologists remove a cell or several cells from the embryo, which are then tested for chromosomal abnormalities.

► **Time Lapse Imaging**

In conventional IVF, the embryologist will check the developing embryos under a microscope, which involves removing them from the incubator for a short period of time. Time-lapse imaging allows them to take thousands of images of the embryos as they grow without disturbing them.

Medicine is developing all the time, so there may be more known about add on procedures when you undergo fertility treatment. These additional treatments have been developed with the intention to improve IVF outcomes, though they may not be proven and they may not help in all cases. With your doctor and your baby-making team, you will need to weigh up these options and the costs to decide if there are treatments you would like to try. Some doctors do not make these available to their patients, whereas others offer them at no cost, so you will need to research what is available at each clinic.

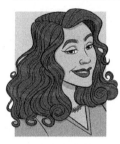

Add ons are largely unproven, though they may have been shown in some studies to be helpful. As long as you're not doing anything harmful and if it might have a chance of helping, why not try it?
- Dr Lynn Burmeister

EXPECTATION VERSUS REALITY

While you must go into IVF hoping that you will be successful, the difficult reality is that you may be stopped at any stage in this process. You may find that you have far fewer embryos than you hoped for. It's typical to lose approximately 50 percent of your embryos at each stage.

For example, you might start with 15 eggs, have 8 fertilise, 4 remaining five days later and only 1 will test PGS Normal.

You may go through the cycle, retrieval, fertilisation and testing process and find that you have no viable embryos at all to transfer.

This is one of the most challenging aspects of fertility treatment. You must somehow go into the process with hope, while at the same time be aware that there is a chance you will not be successful. It is a difficult balance. It is particularly difficult if the members of your baby-making team have different perspectives – perhaps one of you is a glass half full and one is a glass half empty kind of person.

We found that there is no real way to prepare for an unwanted IVF result. Your heart will be broken regardless of whether you go into the process with a lot of hope or just a little. All you can do is have the best possible strategies in place to take care of your mental health and look after your partner if the worst does occur. In most cases, there is something else you can try if you are unsuccessful the first time. And sometimes a new cycle will just bring better luck. Allow yourself to feel your disappointment for a time and then dust yourself off and do whatever you need to do to prepare yourself for the next steps.

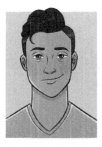

*We wanted two kids. We had two very nice-looking embryos that had been sent off for PGS testing. We were going to transfer them first, but the results were taking a long time to come back. It was frustrating at the time. We decided to start another egg retrieval cycle while we were waiting. Due to this extra cycle, we were lucky enough to end up with a total of four PGS normal embryos. The first transfer failed, and the second became our son. If we hadn't done another cycle before getting pregnant, my wife might have been too old to produce eggs for our second child. Thank goodness we still have frozen embryos ready to try. Sometimes things just work out the way that they're supposed to. - **Chris***

EMBRYO TRANSFER

The next step of an IVF cycle is the transfer, when an embryo is placed back inside the uterus, usually five days after the egg retrieval. Your doctor or embryologist may suggest transferring earlier on the third day after retrieval, ask them to explain why they believe that is the best course of action.

Or, you might be opting to do a Frozen Embryo Transfer (FET), which means you are using a frozen embryo from a previous egg retrieval months or even years before now.

After so much craziness, this part is relatively simple. The person who will carry the pregnancy simply lies back in a chair with their legs in the stirrups and the doctor uses ultrasound and a long catheter to place the embryo into the perfect position. Hopefully, that is where it will stay for the next nine months. This is an important day, so do your very best to be there to hold your partner's hand during the procedure.

Preparing for your Embryo Transfer with **Dr Lynn Burmeister**

► *Be as healthy as possible*

► *Meditate and focus on positive thoughts*

► *Be as relaxed as possible*

► *Acupuncture may help. There are some studies that show it may be beneficial on the day of the transfer.*

► *I don't really think that eating French fries after transfer helps, but some people believe that superstition. If it makes you happy, then that is good.*

► *We know that happiness improves your chance of embryo transfer success, this has been shown in multiple studies. So, go home after your transfer and watch a funny movie, something so ridiculous that you laugh all the way through it.*

► *And finally, know that laughing will not push your embryo out!*

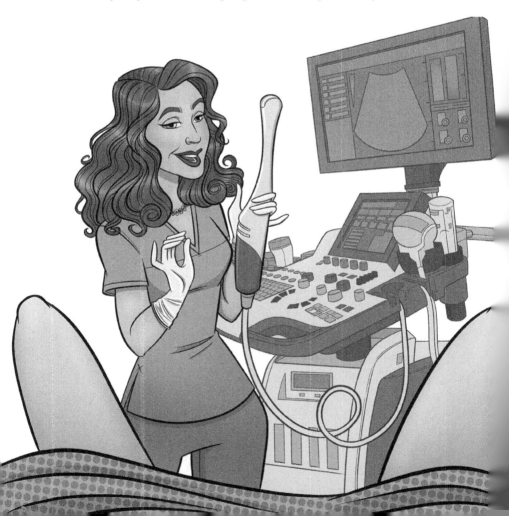

GIFTS, TIPS AND GOOD LUCK CHARMS

Women are usually very connected in to the 'IVF Community'. That means they are reading all the infertility online groups and forums, following all the IVF social media influencers and maybe even meeting up in real life with women from their IVF tribe. Generally, men are not as linked in.

So, we're going to give you some tips that she will most likely already know about. By participating in these superstitions or giving her one of these thoughtful gifts, your partner will feel your genuine caring. Of course, we know you do care, but this will help her feel it. Some of these tips are very strange, but in the uncertain world of fertility treatment, it's best to just go with it, in case it actually works!

IVF got this

Cute expressions and one-liners are a big feature of the IVF community, particularly on social media. A note, message or a gift with one of these phrases on it will be well-received by your partner.

Some common phrases:
- ▶ IVF got this
- ▶ Wake, pray, transfer day
- ▶ Retrieve, believe, conceive
- ▶ Embaby on board
- ▶ Worth every shot
- ▶ IVF Warrior
- ▶ Infertility Warrior
- ▶ Everything crossed but my legs

Laughter

This may seem odd, but there are some studies suggesting women who laugh and relax after embryo transfer are more likely to have success. When you are laughing, you are not stressed. Stress hormones increase heart rate, blood pressure, respiration rate, blood flow to muscles and metabolic rate, which would have been great for facing danger in our cave dweller days. These same hormones shut down reproduction, digestion and growth – systems not needed for the response to an immediate threat. Laughter may make her body more receptive to nurture your tiny embryo. After embryo transfer, have some funny movies on standby and a relaxing afternoon planned.

McDonald's Fries

Don't ask how this superstition got started, nobody knows. People go straight to McDonald's after an embryo transfer to eat fries and many swear that it was the thing that made their IVF cycle successful. Does it have to be McDonald's fries? Yes, apparently it does.

Perhaps it comes from when doctors would recommend eating salty foods after an egg retrieval to prevent ovarian hyperstimulation syndrome (OHSS). Someone shared the story of how Maccas fries got her pregnant and it was passed on and passed on... and a new superstition was born. Over time, it became something to do after embryo transfer and not after egg retrieval... who knows why? Still, it's an opportunity to have some tasty fries and to connect with your partner, so why not?

FROM JON

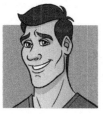

We opted to make some healthier oven baked homemade fries, but if McDonald's fries makes you and your partner feel happy on transfer day, then that has got to be a good thing.

Socks

A widely held principle in Chinese medicine is that a 'cold' uterus or one with poor blood flow and circulation can be a cause of infertility. Some women take the precaution of wearing warm socks throughout an IVF cycle, especially on transfer day, so as not to let heat escape the body. It is hoped that the blood flow will warm up the uterus, rather than being diverted to cold feet. Some warm and comfy socks would be a lovely gift for your partner.

Pineapples

The theory is that pineapple (especially the core) contains something called bromelain. It is a collection of enzymes that help break down and digest food. When taken on an empty stomach, bromelain may act as a blood thinner and an anti-inflammatory, and all of this may help an embryo implant into the uterus.

Now, we've never heard a doctor yell, "GET HER A PINEAPPLE STAT!" or "SHE NEEDS AN IV OF PINA COLADA IMMEDIATELY!" but it's another superstition that can't hurt. So, why not? Get her a couple of pineapples to eat after her embryo transfer or insemination. Any gift with a pineapple print on it will also be a big hit.

Milestone Cards

IVF Milestone Cards are perfect for recording all those important moments on your IVF journey. What is a milestone card, you may ask? It is a piece of card or even wood with a cute expression and when you reach a certain milestone in your IVF journey, you snap a photo while holding the card. They say things like 'First Injection', 'Follicle Scan' or 'Transfer Day'. They might also include motivational statements such as 'IVF Got This' or 'This journey is tough, but so are we'.

Get involved in capturing the moments along the way using milestone cards. With any luck, your infertility journey will have a happy ending and you will want to look back on these memories. And even if the journey doesn't end the way you hope it will, it is still important to acknowledge and remember your resilience throughout your experience.

Elephants

Elephants are pregnant for up to 22 months. They have to wait much longer for their babies than other animals. Remember that scene in the movie Dumbo, where Mrs Dumbo is waiting for the stork? In fact, the elephant has the longest pregnancy of all mammals. It makes sense that the elephant would be a symbol for the infertility community, who seem to always be waiting. Your partner will appreciate any gift with elephants on it. The story below is sometimes shared on the internet and in the IVF community.

Your partner will appreciate any gift with elephants on it. The story below is sometimes shared on the internet and in the IVF community.

An elephant and a dog became pregnant at the same time. Three months down the line, the dog gave birth to six puppies. Six months later, the dog was pregnant again and nine months on it gave birth to another dozen puppies. The pattern continued. During the 18th month the dog approached the elephant questioning,

"Are you sure that you are pregnant? We became pregnant on the same date, I have given birth three times to a dozen puppies and they have now grown to become big dogs, yet you are still pregnant. What's going on?"

The elephant replied, "There is something I want you to understand. What I am carrying is not a puppy, but an elephant. I only give birth to one in two years. When my baby hits the ground, the earth shakes. When my baby crosses the road, human beings stop and watch in admiration. What I'm carrying is mighty and great."

Don't lose faith when you see others receive answers to their prayers. Don't be envious. If you haven't received your own blessings, don't despair. Say to yourself, "My time is coming, and when it hits the surface of the earth, people shall yield in admiration and the ground will shake."

Baby Onesie

Hopefully, your IVF journey will bring you a baby. If you are lucky enough to have a child at the end of your journey, it's nice to acknowledge all that you went through to meet that little person. One way that many choose to do that is with a little onesie with some words relating to how that child came to be. These can be purchased online and have phrases such as 'Made with Love and a Little Science', 'Worth the Wait', 'The Little Embryo that Could' and 'I Survived the Ice Age'. A baby gift with a reference to the infertility that is now behind you would be a lovely gift at the end of your journey.

Go to www.InfertilityMan.com/MansGuide to find infertility themed gifts.

THE TWO-WEEK WAIT

This is an especially challenging part of fertility treatment. After transferring the embryo into the uterus, you face the dreaded 'two-week wait', also known as the TWW. Time will never move more slowly than it does during these weeks. It can be a time of utter insanity. Amongst infertility circles, the woman is now described as PUPO – pregnant until proven otherwise. Some prefer to use the term PASP – pregnant and staying pregnant. It takes about two weeks for the pregnancy hormones to build up in the woman's body so that there is enough there to accurately show pregnancy on a blood or urine test. At this stage, you've done all you can do, it's now in God's or the universe's or anyone else's hands but your own.

So, you wait... and wait... and wait.

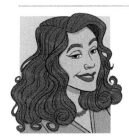

The two-week wait is a really difficult time. I think it's best to keep yourself really busy, don't just lie in bed, don't take time off work, keep yourself occupied. I have heard of people taking a holiday, which is a nice idea. Just try to avoid stress - that's not going to help the embryo stick! - **Dr Lynn Burmeister**

She might be 'symptom spotting' and noticing every little thing that feels different in her body and every little thing that feels the same. She might be peeing on pregnancy tests every single day and squinting at the little lines or she may have banned herself from testing. One minute she is absolutely sure she is pregnant and the next minute she is sure she's not. You suddenly start searching online for anything to give you hope. Then you realise it's making you more stressed so you ban yourself from the internet. You wonder if you're going insane. It feels like the longest two weeks in all eternity.

The best thing you can do is to keep yourself busy and your mind relaxed. It's recommended that she keeps her body from overheating, so limit strenuous exercise. If you want to do something to help with implantation, then healthy food, good rest and lots of water is all you can do.

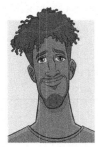

We had lots of ups and downs along the way, even with just the usual things that happen during an IVF cycle. The five-day wait and then after the five-day wait you've got the two week wait where you're waiting for PGD results and then waiting for the right day of her cycle and then an embryo transfer and then another two week wait. There is a lot of waiting and that is challenging in itself. - Lamar

Tip: Be careful with home pregnancy tests when undergoing fertility treatment. Be aware that sometimes fertility medications can give you a false positive. And testing too early can give you a false negative. Many women who are trying to conceive will test every day in their two-week wait, which could make anyone feel crazy. They will write on each stick how many days past the transfer they are (for example 6DP5DT, 6 days past 5-day transfer) and compare the intensity of the little faint lines. Decide with your baby-making team what you plan to do regarding home pregnancy testing and stick to that.

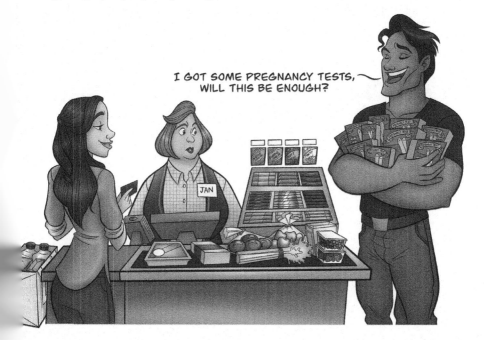

PREGNANCY TESTS

Your fertility clinic will have a plan for you to find out the results of your fertility treatment. Somewhere close to 11 days after your transfer, she will have a blood test and get a phone call to confirm if she is pregnant or not. Whatever the result, be sure that your schedule is clear, you will want to be there to receive the news. If it's good news, you will want to celebrate and if it's not you will need to be there to support each other and process your own emotions.

It's a Big Fat Negative (BFN)

There are so many ways that an IVF cycle can fail, and often they do. A BFN might happen for several reasons.

▶ There were no eggs to collect.

▶ There was no sperm available.

▶ There were eggs, but they didn't fertilise.

▶ They didn't grow into blastocysts.

▶ Embryos didn't survive the freezing/thawing process.

▶ An embryo was transferred, but it didn't take.

▶ It does take but it doesn't stick around, resulting in a chemical pregnancy or an early pregnancy loss.

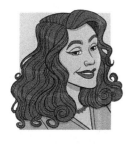

Unfortunately, not every IVF cycle is going to be successful, we know that. Most of the time, the statistics are against you. The chance of a negative result is higher than the chance of a positive result. It does depend on your age and your circumstance. After an unsuccessful cycle, your doctor should go through everything with you, so make sure that they have done every investigation that may provide answers. They may do tests to see if there is something wrong with implantation or the implantation window. They might test to see if they can find autoimmune issues. Most often, the cause lies with the embryo or with embryo quality. The most likely reason that an embryo doesn't implant is the embryo itself. Be gentle with yourself after an unsuccessful cycle. **- Dr Lynn Burmeister**

A failed IVF cycle carries with it genuine grief. One thing that certainly hinders the grieving process is the feeling that you have no right to grieve something that was never real. The grief is very real even if a pregnancy didn't begin.

Your partner may really feel this grief, so you should be present in case she needs to vent, talk or wallow. Allow her this time and eventually help her to move forward again.

Remember, it is important to acknowledge your own feelings too. Many men feel like they don't have the right to be sad because the loss didn't physically happen to them. This loss definitely did happen to you. You must take some time to process it in your own way.

Every reproductive loss is different, so the intensity of your response may vary. For information about significant losses, see the chapter later in this book.

If you are experiencing a setback, acknowledge your disappointment, check in to see how your partner is feeling and then do what you need to do to move forward to your next steps in a healthy way.

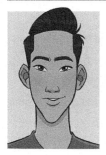 *Whilst it was brutal going through that many cycles, I went in every time believing that this cycle could be the one... in a rational way, not just with blind hope. And I also had the expectation that even if we're not lucky this time, so long as she had it in her to try again and I've got it in me to be there to help her, then we'll keep going for as long as we can keep going.* - **James**

It's a Big Fat Positive (BFP)

Congratulations! We are so happy for you!

BETA HCG LEVELS

Human chorionic gonadotropin, or hCG, is a pregnancy hormone produced by cells around an embryo to help form the placenta. This is the hormone detected by both urine and blood pregnancy tests. The level of hCG can vary a lot from one pregnancy to another, even for the same person. In most cases, you need to see the numbers consistently rising for the first few months of pregnancy before declining again later. In the first four weeks of a viable pregnancy, hCG levels will typically double about every two to three days.

Unfortunately, not all pregnancies continue to a live birth. Many miscarriages take place before the woman even knows she is pregnant. When you get pregnant through fertility treatment, you will know you're pregnant very early. Your fertility clinic will perform several blood tests in the first two weeks after you receive a positive result to make sure that the HCG levels are rising appropriately.

FROM JON

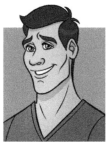

We transferred an embryo and were amazed to learn that it had worked – we were pregnant. We did a home pregnancy test and then a blood test at the clinic confirmed the good news. Finally, after three years and so many procedures, we were pregnant. We felt relieved, excited and overjoyed... but the overwhelming feeling was disbelief – how had we suddenly become so lucky? Laura's first hCG level was 200, so we were off to a flying start.

We celebrated and took our time to adjust to the new reality. We watched the little video of our embryo being fertilised in the lab with tears in our eyes, so excited that this little embryo was the one that was going to make it. Little did we know that the first few weeks of this pregnancy would be some of our most challenging yet.

Two days later, Laura returned to the clinic for a second blood test. Laura was feeling extra tired, so she was having long naps, certain in the idea that she needed to take care of herself to protect this brand-new life. That afternoon, we received a call from the nurse with the news that the hCG level was not rising as we needed it to. This news hit us like a tonne of bricks. The nurse was concerned and told us that now was the time to be strong. She booked us to come back in two days for another blood test.

We tried to stay positive and prayed that this baby would stick around. Laura's mind was racing, she was rationalising, pleading and negotiating with the universe. She was already mapping out in her calendar what it would look like if she had to do another IVF cycle and figuring out how long she would need to recover from an early miscarriage. She was exhausted and slept for long periods. She was physically and emotionally drained.

That Friday, Laura went in for yet another blood test. We really needed to see an improvement in the hCG numbers this time. Waiting for the call that afternoon was pretty stressful, we both jumped every time the phone rang. The nurse confirmed the worst; the hCG had not risen enough.

Laura asked the nurse to be honest with us. "Do you ever see pregnancies with these hCG numbers continue?" The nurse answered that she had never seen that happen. She had arranged an ultrasound on Monday so we could see what was happening inside Laura's uterus and decide the next steps. We would have to wait through the entire weekend to find out what was going on.

The next few days were some of the most difficult that we had both lived through. Laura developed a sharp pain in the left side of her stomach. She felt like the pain was in her ovary or her fallopian tube. She wondered if this was a developing ectopic pregnancy. She was extremely tired and spent the two days in bed. In Laura's mind, the pregnancy was over. She needed to come to terms with it and she felt like it was better to accept that the baby wasn't there anymore before seeing it on the scan on Monday. I knew Laura needed to feel this, but I hated to see her so upset.

The best way I knew how to support her was to bring her food and water, listen to whatever she had to tell me, and hold her when she cried. We hadn't told anyone else about what we were going through, so it was just the two of us. It was difficult for me to process my own feelings of loss while at the same time being strong enough to comfort her. I wanted to be strong for her, but I was also losing this pregnancy and it hurt.

The hours ticked by so slowly as we counted down to our ultrasound. Finally, it was time. We were both relieved to be finally getting some answers but at the same time dreading the news that we were both certain would be negative. I wasn't going to let her go through this alone. When we approached the receptionist, she could see it in my face that I was coming in, no matter what.

The silence was deafening in that tiny room. Laura was too upset to even look at the ultrasound screen. I was watching intently when I saw a little flicker. The sonographer, who we had gotten to know quite well during our treatment, breathed a sigh of relief.

"There is a little heartbeat."

This was one of those moments in life when everything stands still and your ears don't hear what is happening around you. My eyes focused in on that little flickering heartbeat. The sonographer was trying to explain to Laura that the baby was still alive, but Laura couldn't process the information. She kept shaking her head. I snapped out of it to help her understand.

"There's a heartbeat."

It was good news and it was emotionally overwhelming. It could have very easily been a totally different outcome.

The sonographer moved the ultrasound to look at Laura's left ovary. It was swollen to about 20 times the usual size, probably due to the stress we had put it under doing many back-to-back IVF cycles over the past 12 months. That explained the pain she had been feeling.

This experience early in the pregnancy changed our approach to the entire nine months. We took more time before telling family and friends and we didn't share anything online until the pregnancy was 32 weeks along. I guess we never really felt certain that everything was ok, even though the rest of the pregnancy was very normal and uneventful.

This is our story. We were very lucky that this embryo transfer continued into a healthy pregnancy. We don't want to give false hope. Most often, pregnancies with slow rising hCG levels do not continue. We want you to be aware that a positive pregnancy test might still result in a chemical pregnancy or an early miscarriage. At the same time, nothing is really over until you have the definitive results. Keep hope alive, stay balanced and take care of each other. This journey is a crazy ride. It will certainly require all the strength you have.

That tiny flickering light ended up becoming our daughter.

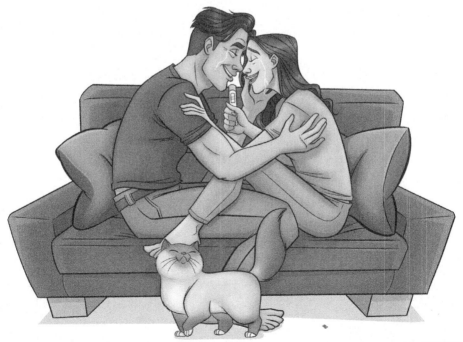

BABY-MAKING MEET UP

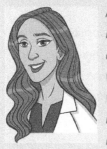

My best advice for supporting your partner during IVF is to discuss it in advance. Set aside time to answer questions like:

What do I need during the cycle?

What do YOU need during the cycle?

How can we communicate with each other?

How can we celebrate small wins together - doing the first shots, making it to the egg retrieval, doing an embryo transfer?

- Dr Lora Shahine

Hormones

Discuss in advance the plan in case the hormones make her a little crazy. Ask her how she would like you to take care of her in those moments. It might be making her a cup of tea, giving her a hug or a massage or reminding her it's ok to take a nap. If you have agreed on some strategies in advance, then when she is feeling particularly hormonal, she will be reminded that you care when you offer up one of these ideas. The rational part of her brain that is still there under all those fertility medications will remember this conversation and she will hopefully feel your good intentions.

Injections

How would she like to be helped with her injections? Do you have the protocol and the medications you need? Do you need to pick anything up from the pharmacy?

Ultrasounds and Retrieval

Does she want you to come with her to these appointments? Have you got the things she would like to help recover after the retrieval, for example, a heat pack, warm socks, and chocolate?

If you are having sperm retrieval surgery, what do you need to do to support yourself before and after your procedure?

Fertilisation and Testing

What is the plan for fertilisation? Will you make all the eggs into embryos before freezing or just some? Will you opt for pre-implantation genetic testing?

Transfer

Are you hoping to do a fresh embryo transfer or freezing all? What is your plan for transfer day? How would she like to be supported? Which funny movie would you like to watch together?

The Two-Week Wait

How will you manage the emotions of the Two-Week Wait? How will you distract yourselves? How would she like to be supported?

Unexpected Outcomes

Talk a little about what you hope will happen during the cycle. How will you manage if it doesn't go according to plan?

AFTER FERTILITY TREATMENT

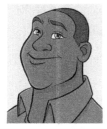

We had 'the chat.' The doctor said to us 'IVF doesn't work for everybody. I will continue to treat you as I don't believe it's completely futile yet, but please know that I don't know if this will work for you.' She was trying to let us know we were nearly at the point of wasting our time. **- Terrence**

When your fertility treatment does not result in a pregnancy, it can be very upsetting. Whether you were logically expecting it to work or even if you believe success was unlikely, it still hurts.

It brings up so many questions:

▶ Should you try again?

▶ Should you to move to a different type of fertility treatment?

▶ How do you decide when it is time to stop fertility treatment?

▶ Should you look at other pathways to parenthood?

▶ How do you come to the decision to remain childless?

The answers you seek are not simple and only you can decide for yourself.

When you don't get the outcome you desire, it may be tempting to simply rush into more fertility treatment. However, it is at this point that you need to exercise a bit of patience. First, your bodies may need time to heal and replenish, as may your mind and your soul. Give yourself time to reflect, to process what you have been through. Allow your partner (or baby-making team) the time, space and support that they need to feel their way through the grief that inevitably comes with failed treatment.

▶ Is your mental health suffering?

▶ Do you no longer feel like your 'old self'?

▶ Is it getting more and more difficult to front up to the fertility clinic?

▶ Is it impacting on your financial stability?

▶ Is it affecting your mood day-to-day?

- Is it affecting your relationship?
- Do you often feel you have little or no energy?
- Do you feel flat, grumpy and out of sorts?
- Is it affecting your friendships or your work?
- Have you put on hold major decisions, such as moving house, changing jobs, travel, study or other important life plans because you are waiting to get pregnant?

These are possibly signs that it is time to stop. Or maybe it is time to take a break and have a rest from fertility treatment for a period of time. Perhaps you need to seek some professional support or counselling. Take some time to regain some sense of normality in order to make these big decisions.

If you consider The 7 Mindsets of Infertility, where are you right now? Where is your partner?

THE 7 MINDSETS OF INFERTILITY

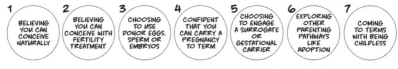

Many people get stuck in a mindset that realistically may never give them the outcome they desire. They might get stuck doing the same thing over and over again, getting no closer to their end goal. Sometimes miracles happen on the sixth or the fifteenth IVF round, but this may be unlikely in your case. And sometimes the miracle happens when you open your heart to new possibilities and perhaps a new pathway to parenthood. Only you can know the right way forward for you.

- Does your current mindset serve you?
- Would it be intelligent to move to a different one?
- When would be a good time to make the decision?

At some point, it may become clear that conceiving with fertility treatment is not the way forward for you. Perhaps a doctor has recommended that you try something different, as your own eggs, sperm or uterus is just not going to create and sustain a pregnancy. Perhaps you have tried so many times through several IVF cycles or miscarriages and you just don't have it in you to keep trying anymore. You might be physically, financially and emotionally drained, and it's time to consider a different way forward.

▶ And in that case, which mindset would be most beneficial for you right now?
▶ How does your partner feel about that?
▶ How can you both reach a mindset that is the best possible choice for you both, under the circumstances?

FROM JON

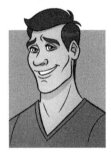

A wise fella told me once that you become a dad long before you become a dad. I asked what he meant, and he talked about setting the example of a man you would want to be as a role model for your children. You can begin that evolution before you become a father, in fact, that is the best way.

Regardless of where you are on your fertility journey at this moment in time, you can keep working to be the man that you would like to be for your family in the future. Regardless of whether you conceive a child, choose other paths to parenthood or remain childless, you can still be a role model. It is more to do with how you show up in your life for the people you care about than how many children you have.

PATHS TO PARENTHOOD

EGG, SPERM AND EMBRYO DONATION

Depending on your infertility diagnosis, donation may be a good choice for you. Donor sperm can fertilise your partner's eggs, or donor eggs can be used with your sperm. Or you could choose donated embryos. Embryo donation often involves IVF patients donating their unused embryos. The embryos are then transferred into the uterus to hopefully begin a pregnancy.

▶ How will you feel about having a child who is not biologically yours?
▶ How will you select a donor?
▶ How will you tell your child about how they were conceived?

These are just some of the important questions to ask yourself and your baby-making team, if you decide to move on to Mindset 3 and use donor conception in the hope of building your family.

A big consideration is that one or both of the intended parents will lose their genetic connection to the child. For some, parenting is more about forming a loving bond with a child, not so much about seeing their genetics play out in that child. For others, it's a massive hurdle to overcome. It is perfectly understandable to feel a sense of grief about not having a biological link to your child. It may take time to overcome these feelings. Same-sex couples always face this challenge, and the same emotional obstacles may still apply. Donor conception has lifelong implications for the child, who may seek to know where they come from, potentially making a connection with their donor parents or with their biological siblings out in the world.

There are many emotional, legal, physical and financial aspects for you to consider before going down the road of donor conception. Many families report that donor conception is an incredibly beautiful experience and does not make any difference to their sense of love and connection to their child.

Finding a Donor

The task of finding egg, sperm or embryo donors can certainly be challenging.

In some countries, donation of eggs, sperm or embryos must be altruistic, which means that you can't pay someone for their donation. In other places, egg, sperm and embryo banks exist where donors can be paid.

Donation Options

► Asking someone you know, often a sibling, cousin, relative or friend.
► Linking with a donor through your fertility clinic.
► Advertising for a donor in print media or on a relevant website.
► Travelling overseas where donor banks are available or agencies that connect donors with recipients.

Your IVF clinic should be able to provide you with information and advice about finding donors. Sperm donation is physically easier to provide, whereas a female providing eggs will need to go through an IVF egg retrieval and all the associated medications and surgery.

You will need to consider:

► What is motivating this person (or these people) to want to donate?
► How old they are?
► Do they have children already?
► Are they physically and mentally healthy?
► Are they happy to be identified to the child when they are older?

If you are heading overseas, find out in advance how you will choose your donor and what information you can learn about them. This will help with your decision-making. Arrangements overseas can be very different, so find out all you can in advance.

The Process

Donors should undergo extensive medical screening processes, including checks for things like hepatitis, cystic fibrosis, syphilis, chlamydia and HIV. Blood group tests allow your doctor to know of any potential issues between the embryo and the woman who will carry the pregnancy.

Counselling is a necessary step before donation, for both you and your partner (if applicable). If using a known donor, they will also need to attend counselling along with their partner, if they have one. It's an important part of preparing for donor conception and it will cause you to think through many ideas and scenarios that you might not have considered. It's important to fully understand what you are all getting into. Also, it is very important for the donor to truly understand what they will be putting their body through, along with the legal and emotional implications of having a biological child out in the world with another family.

Donor relationships can be created through family members, for example, your wife may receive a donor egg from her sister. They have had a lifetime to get to know each other. It is important that both of their partners have the opportunity to establish and understand their own relationships, which is why the counselling is so important. Also, if you will have an ongoing relationship with your donor, they need to clearly understand their relationship with the child and not overstep any boundaries with your parenting style.

Make sure that your counsellor is a good fit for you and that they are helping you to address the important issues (if not, don't be afraid to find a new one). The conversations might be awkward, but they are vital to address all the issues which have the potential to become bigger problems down the track. Don't feel the need to be agreeable or on 'good behaviour' just because you want the donation to go ahead. It is far more important to be honest to ensure that the donor relationship will work well, which is better for you, your donor, and any potential children.

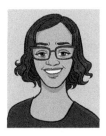

It really is important to access your own mental health support. You need to process your grief before jumping into donor conception or surrogacy. Get counselling as a couple, but also on your own, just because you need it. Talk through whatever is coming up, there is no right or wrong. If you're feeling something like 'I'm angry that I won't have a genetic connection to my child,' - just feel it, talk about it, access some support and discuss it with someone qualified. Make sure that you are not dumping it onto your partner or your surrogate – because they are processing their own emotions too.

- Sarah Jefford, Family Creation Lawyer (Surrogacy & Donor Conception)

Legal

Obviously, donor conception is subject to the laws of your location and pertains to the rights of the donors, the intended parents and the child. Look carefully into the legalities of when a donor can withdraw consent. Usually it is up until such time that the eggs, sperm or embryos are used in fertilisation, or once they are inserted into the uterus.

The birth certificate will give legal parental rights to the recipient parents, including the responsibility to provide for the child. Donors hand over all custodial rights from the moment that the embryo is created or the pregnancy begins.

Costs

Costs vary greatly depending on your location and if you are purchasing the genetic matter. Even if you are receiving altruistically from a known donor, you will be expected to cover their medical bills and any other reasonable costs, such as travel.

Some countries may provide rebates for donor IVF cycles, so look to see if you can claim. Then there are the usual IVF costs on top of that, plus any legal fees associated with setting up the agreement.

As with all infertility treatment, using donor eggs, sperm or embryos does not guarantee a pregnancy or live birth, though it may significantly increase your chances. Consider your likelihood of success against the potential costs and decide if donor conception is the right choice for you.

Emotional Considerations

Sometimes, men can find the concept of using donor sperm difficult. Perhaps it is to do with the idea of family legacy and passing on your own genetics. Women can also find egg donation difficult, though if they are able to carry the pregnancy themselves, then at least they have a physical connection to the child in a way that men obviously cannot.

With time and counselling, most men are able to overcome these concerns, with the prospect of a family being the most important outcome. So, make sure you reach out to get the support you need. You might find it best to chat to a mate, someone who has been through infertility or donor conception before or a professional. Finding men who share their infertility story online can also be a big help, as can support groups.

If you are unable to provide sperm to get your partner pregnant, the next best thing you can do is to take the necessary steps to be in a good mindset in order to use donor sperm. Many men report feeling concerned about letting go of their genetic link initially, but once their children are born, they deem it to be unimportant and they love their children with an instant bond.

Our journey to parenthood took 12 years, we eventually had our child using 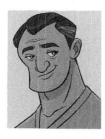 *donor eggs. I definitely grieved the genetic loss. I wanted our child to have my wife's blue eyes and beautiful smile. It was hard to let go of little things like that. But, now that we actually have him, I couldn't imagine it any differently. If his genetics were different, then he wouldn't be him, and I would never want to change him. My son's existence makes so much of that difficult journey worthwhile. It's completely in the past. - **Brendan**

SURROGACY

Surrogacy is where a woman carries a pregnancy for another person or couple. Should your partner not be able to carry a pregnancy or if you don't have a female partner, then surrogacy might be an option for you.

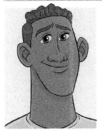

Before I needed it, I hadn't put that much thought into what surrogacy was. I had a plan in my mind for how my family was going to be made, and that was that. Counselling helped me to change my ideas and come to terms with the new plan. I found out you actually have quite a lot of options. **- Alex**

Much of the information about surrogacy is centred around women, as they are the ones who will be pregnant or who are processing the idea of not being able to carry their own baby. While you play a very important role in supporting your partner and the surrogate, it is important to remember that you are experiencing this as well. You will have your own emotions to process and you will need to prepare yourself for this challenging and beautiful way of building your family.

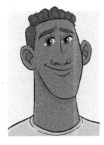

The journey of surrogacy is centred around the women which makes sense as pregnancy is a female thing. Men can be a little neglected. At our first fertility appointments, my wife and the doctor were speaking so fast, I could barely get a word in. As time went on, if there was something that I felt was important, I would say, 'stop for a second'. I really wanted to be as involved as I could. **- Alex**

There are many situations that draw people into a surrogacy arrangement:

▶ A same sex couple wanting children.

▶ A man choosing to be a single parent.

▶ A woman or couple who can't carry a pregnancy due to medical reasons.

Whatever your situation, there is likely to be a sense of grief that you will work through as you adjust your image of how pregnancy will be in your life. Your partner may feel disappointed that she doesn't get to be pregnant and birth her child herself. You might feel some sadness about not being able to cuddle up to the baby bump at night, to feel all those little kicks and play the doting partner during the pregnancy. It is vital that you prepare yourself emotionally and mentally, which is why counselling, both with your partner and on your own, is so important.

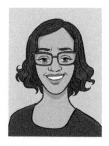

So much of the support is geared towards women. The male partner usually spends a lot of his energy in that supportive role; it's all about her. It is hard to work out what these intended fathers need. Most of the time, the men don't even know and they tend not to talk. Men need support too. Many of them have a dream of their partner being pregnant with their baby and growing their family. They have to adjust that dream to accept that somebody else is going to carry their child. There is a grief that goes along with that. And it's not just the woman's grief, the men feel it too. - Sarah Jefford, Family Creation Lawyer (Surrogacy & Donor Conception)

The Process

Surrogacy is a very involved process that will require lots of forethought and preparation. Once again, the process and laws regarding surrogacy will be different depending on your location and situation.

Counselling will involve talking through issues with all parties separately and together to help prepare for surrogacy. It is important to be honest during this phase, rather than trying to say the 'right' thing. You need to be truthful in order to identify and address issues now rather than later, when they may be harder to fix. It is a huge decision for someone to offer to be a surrogate, just as it is incredibly challenging for intended parents, hoping to grow their family through surrogacy.

An assessment will be carried out which, although conducted by a counsellor, psychologist or psychiatrist, is different from the general counselling sessions. It is a more formal process to assess the motivation and suitability of all parties in the surrogacy proposal. The process is extensive and is set up to ensure that the decisions made are in the best interests of the child and all parties.

Once the surrogacy agreement has been reached, then the IVF process can begin. Trying to conceive in this way has the same highs and lows of any fertility treatment, there are just more of you involved. Be prepared that it may not go to plan; the success rates are the same, although your chances may be improved on where you were before.

It is an incredibly difficult decision to ask someone to be a surrogate, as it will definitely impact on their life and even on their health. While surrogacy can be a beautiful gift, it can have serious implications for the surrogate and her family, so it needs to be carefully considered. It can also be deeply rewarding for all parties and can have beautiful outcomes.

Legal

The laws about surrogacy are dependent on your location and they are updated and changed all the time. They stipulate who can access surrogacy and under what conditions. Some places require you to be in a marriage or marriage-like relationship for a certain period of time, others have no such requirement. Some places still make surrogacy illegal, even if you travel overseas to access it.

There will certainly be legal hoops to jump through, and both the intended parents and the surrogate will need separate lawyers who specialise in surrogacy agreements.

A surrogate may have to meet requirements such as:
▶ Being medically and psychologically suitable.
▶ Being within certain age restrictions.
▶ Having children of their own already.
▶ Having had no previous pregnancy complications.
▶ Only performing a single embryo transfer.

The regulations and psychological support are in place to prevent an arrangement where the surrogate becomes too attached and feels unable to hand over the baby. The aim is to ensure that all parties are protected from unwanted outcomes, but the rules do make surrogacy an incredibly difficult area to navigate. Be aware of the point at which parties can no longer change their mind and make sure that you are ok with that arrangement. Having a written agreement in place serves the important purpose of making each person consider their expectations about how the relationship will work, as well as the rights of any children produced.

The agreement will cover more immediate concerns, such as:
▶ Who is responsible for the medical costs and other expenses?
▶ Who will select medical carers?
▶ How will the surrogate behave during the pregnancy, for example, what she should eat or drink.
▶ Who will attend the birth?
▶ How involved can the intended parents be during pregnancy?
▶ What happens in the event of miscarriage or stillbirth?
▶ What happens if the intended parents die or separate?

Costs

Even when surrogacy is provided without payment to the surrogate, the costs can be substantial. You will need to cover all reasonable costs of the surrogate, such as medical, travel and even lost wages. In addition to the cost of fertility treatment, the legal costs should also be included in your budget.

Going Overseas

As with embryo, egg or sperm donation, some people choose to go overseas where surrogacy may be easier to access. Some countries only allow altruistic surrogacy, whereas in others payment to the surrogate is allowed. It is not well regulated in some places and there are valid concerns about the exploitation of women in such arrangements.

You will need to consider the laws of the country you are considering getting surrogacy from, as well as ensuring you can get a parenting order and citizenship for any child born overseas. Get good legal advice and ensure you are using a reputable service provider that has your and the surrogate's best interests in mind. You will need to carefully weigh up the ethics and expenses of any surrogacy arrangement, remembering that there is no guarantee of success.

Emotional Considerations

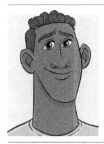 *I missed the usual parts of pregnancy, like getting to feel the baby kick and all that sort of stuff. I must have had a calming energy because the few times I got to put my hand on the surrogate's tummy, there was nothing, hardly a single movement - but it was still amazing to experience. - **Alex***

Surrogacy can be a beautiful way to build your family, and it can be hugely challenging emotionally. It is difficult for women who either have to watch someone else carry their child or who have to give back a child they have carried. It is challenging for men too, there is a grief about not seeing your partner pregnant or having the birth of your child happen the way you thought it would. It can be even more emotionally complex if there is an unexpected outcome, such as pregnancy loss.

Having a baby is a very intimate event in your life. It can be difficult to let go of the idea of how you thought it was going to happen. Surrogacy can bring about unexpected feelings of jealousy, even in otherwise happy arrangements. Couples, gay and straight, can feel an underlying resentment about the fact that they need to invite other people, including lawyers and counsellors, into an experience that they would have preferred to share in private with their partner.

Intended parents don't get to experience the mundanities of pregnancy up close, the morning sickness, getting up to pee 20 times in the night, running out to buy pregnancy craving foods. Some intended parents could be blindsided because the physical presence of the baby is not there until after the birth, which can be a big adjustment.

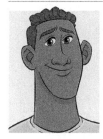

The highlight for me was being able to be there for the birth. I got to have the first skin-to-skin contact, our surrogate did not want to hold the baby immediately after the birth. She was nervous about forming a bond with the baby, she fought that the whole way through. - Alex

It is so important that each person accesses support and counselling so they can resolve any concerns without making it harder for anyone else involved in the surrogacy agreement. If you do the emotional work and step into your surrogacy arrangement with love and caring, it can be a beautiful way to have a baby. And what a lucky child to arrive in the world, already so very loved.

Tip: During pregnancy, the baby comes to know the voices of the parents because they hear them from about 18 weeks into the pregnancy. Record your voices reading a book or singing songs and ask your surrogate if she would play the recording to her bump. There are even specialised speakers that gently adhere to her tummy.

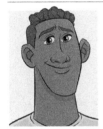

The experience of surrogacy was absolutely amazing. How your child comes into the world doesn't make a difference. Your child is your child and you will love them no matter what. - **Alex**

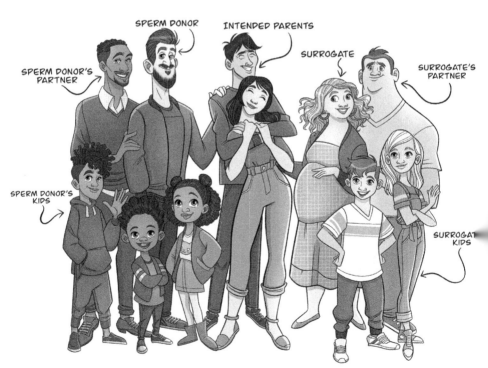

ADOPTION

Adoption permanently transfers the parental rights and responsibilities of biological parents over to adoptive parents.

Moving into the adoption mindset is a considerable undertaking. When people say, "Why don't you just adopt?" to infertile people, they are ill informed about how difficult it can be to access adoption. There are usually only a small number of children who need a new family and they will often have particular needs. It is a very personal decision, but if you (and your partner if applicable) choose to pursue adoption, it could be a beautiful way to build your family.

Eligibility can vary depending on your location, and thankfully, more diverse parental structures are now being accepted than in the past. Couples, single people, same-sex and gender diverse couples are usually welcome, when that may not have previously been the case.

You will need to have a readiness to adopt, meaning that your home, relationship and family are set up to welcome a child into your life. Be aware that you may not be considered suitable if you have a child under the age of one, or if you are pursuing fertility treatment, surrogacy, or if you become pregnant. You may be required to commit to an open adoption, meaning ongoing contact between the adopted child and the biological family.

Again, significant preparation will be required to ensure the preparedness of all parties. Paperwork, counselling, home visits and long conversations are important to ensure that you are all ready for the requirements of building a family in this way. If you feel that adoption is calling you, it could be an incredible way to create your family and give love to a special child.

TELLING YOUR CHILD

When and how to tell your child about how they were born and how they came to be in your family is up to you, and it also depends on the laws within your country. In some places, any child has the right to access information about how they came to be when they reach adulthood and sometimes before.

When going into a donor, surrogacy, or adoption arrangement, be aware of your responsibilities and the rights of your child. Anonymous information may be kept by the state or records may be maintained by your fertility clinic or adoption agency, but it may still be difficult to access information in the future. Find out in advance what happens to all the information, so you are clear on what might happen years later. Of course, if you use a donor or surrogate who you know, they are likely to be in your life in an ongoing way, so you will have an understanding directly with them about how your child will come to know about their biological origins.

In previous generations, children were often not told that their parents were not their biological parents. Research and anecdotal evidence has since proven that this method is not in the best interests of the child. Secrets can be a real burden within families, they can breakdown trust and create unintended feelings of betrayal. Families are created in so many different ways and less conventional family dynamics are becoming more common. Telling your child the truth about where they came from as they grow up can make it less of a shock later in life, although it is never too late to tell.

There are a number of reasons knowing where we come from is important:

▶ Knowing our genetic history can be medically useful, especially regarding inherited diseases.
▶ Our sense of identity and even our mental health can be strongly connected to truthful connections to our heritage.
▶ DNA and blood typing can show when two people are not related, so people can find out even if their parents don't tell them.

▶ There is a potential risk that two people related by blood could form a sexual relationship if they don't know how they were conceived. Knowing their biological heritage could prevent offspring between people sharing common ancestry.

It is recommended to start the conversation while your child is still young so that it's not such a shock when they're old enough to understand. There are children's books available on the topic of donor conception, surrogacy and adoption.

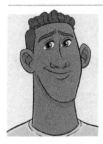

*We have told our boy about how he was conceived since long before he could talk. He has a photo of the surrogacy team up on his bedroom wall. - **Alex***

The greatest journey you will ever embark on

There is obviously so much to understand about these paths to parenthood, so much more than we could include here. If you begin a journey into embryo, egg or sperm donation, surrogacy or adoption, this is just the beginning. We encourage you to seek out information, counselling and support that will help you manage the challenges and create a beautiful parenting experience.

BABY-MAKING MEET UP

If you or your partner is considering one of these alternative paths to parenthood, you will need to have many conversations to decide if it is the right path for you.

First, you must come to a place where you and your partner (if applicable) agree and are in the same mindset. If you are considering a different way of building your family, it might be time to invite new people on to your baby-making team.

THE 7 MINDSETS OF INFERTILITY

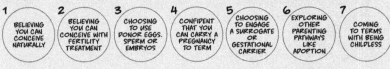

1	2	3	4	5	6	7
BELIEVING YOU CAN CONCEIVE NATURALLY	BELIEVING YOU CAN CONCEIVE WITH FERTILITY TREATMENT	CHOOSING TO USE DONOR EGGS, SPERM OR EMBRYOS	CONFIDENT THAT YOU CAN CARRY A PREGNANCY TO TERM	CHOOSING TO ENGAGE A SURROGATE OR GESTATIONAL CARRIER	EXPLORING OTHER PARENTING PATHWAYS LIKE ADOPTION	COMING TO TERMS WITH BEING CHILDLESS

▶ Which mindset are you all in now?

▶ If you are not in the same mindset as each other, discuss your thoughts and feelings about how you see it differently.

▶ Who do you need to invite on to your team?

▶ How will you approach those conversations?

Building a family using donor eggs, sperm or embryos, using a surrogate or adoption will require you to access professional services.

▶ What research do you need to do?

▶ Where will you connect with services as you move forward down this pathway to parenthood?

▶ Who can help you process your thoughts and feelings?

EXPERIENCING LOSS

FROM LAURA

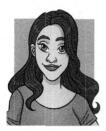

Our daughter was about 11 months old when we decided we should start trying to have a second child. It had been a glorious 18 months of no IVF, no injections and no infertility stress. We had a wonderful straight-forward pregnancy, an amazing birth and a lovely year enjoying our first baby. We felt so 'normal'; just like any other young family. It was difficult to face the fact that we would need to go through fertility treatment all over again if we wanted to grow our family.

It was time. Time to get back in the trenches and face it all again. I was 39, so we didn't want to leave it too long. We thought we would be ok this time. We knew what lay ahead of us and we had learnt so much the first time around. We naively thought we had somehow 'beaten' male factor infertility and it would be easier the second time around. It was not.

We are lucky enough to have 9 embryos and 4 straws of sperm in the freezer from the 15 cycles it took to create our daughter. We had two PGS normal embryos, graded 6AB and 5BB; and we had 7 untested embryos, two graded 5AB, one 5CC, one 3BB, one 3BC and two graded 3CC. We also had four straws of frozen sperm.

These numbers and letters are the 'scores' that our embryologist gave the embryos based on how they look. It is similar to school grades, with 'A' being the best and so on. The higher the number, the more developed they are. 'PGS Normal' means that those embryos were able to undergo Pre-implantation Genetic Screening to confirm they had the correct number of chromosomes (we had two PGS abnormal embryos which were discarded). The untested embryos were not hatching in a way that made it possible to PGS test them.

The four straws of sperm were considered low quality with less than a million sperm and only one or two of them in each straw actually twitching. The embryologist told us that after defrosting the sperm, they only use twitching sperm to inject into eggs using the ICSI procedure.

As anyone who has any experience with IVF understands, having nine embryos in the freezer certainly does not mean nine babies. It doesn't even guarantee one baby.

IVF is brutal and people lose more often than they win.

It was difficult because there is a certain peace to knowing that our embryos and sperm were safe in the freezer. It was scary to take them out and try to use them, because we knew we would most certainly lose some of them. This is the most we would ever have and we couldn't make more.

A boat is safe in the harbour, but that is not what boats are made for. An embryo, egg or sperm is safe in the freezer, but that is not what they are made for. It was time to take that leap of faith... again.

I decided I wanted to try to retrieve some more eggs before transferring an embryo back into my uterus to hopefully start a pregnancy. I thought maybe we could use up the frozen sperm and get a couple more embryos. As I was nearly 40 I knew I would be running out of quality eggs. As you can see in our online videos, the cycle didn't go well. It was incredibly challenging trying to manage breastfeeding while doing an egg collection cycle. We were only about to get two eggs from that cycle.

Jon sat me down after my surgery and asked me to stop doing egg collection cycles. He told me it was difficult for him to watch me going through such a painful experience over and over again. He believed we had enough embryos in the freezer for our family and we should stop trying to make more. I reluctantly agreed, relieved that I could give my body a rest from the relentless repetition of IVF cycles.

We prepared to transfer our best embryo the next month. My diet was perfect. I meditated every day and made sure I got plenty of sleep. Our embryo was almost perfect, PGS normal and graded as 6AB, which meant it was already hatching out of its zona pellucida, ready to implant. My uterus lining was perfect. Thick and fluffed up and ready to receive the embryo. We were ready.

The day after the embryo transfer, I started vomiting. My sense of smell intensified. I had tender breasts. I had been pregnant before and I knew the signs. I immediately knew that I was pregnant. The embryo had definitely implanted, and I was pregnant. Jon and I were overjoyed. We were planning to wait for our blood test, but Jon was going away for work, so we decided to do a home pregnancy test before he left. Two lines confirmed I was indeed pregnant.

It was a perfect embryo, and we knew from the testing that it had the correct number of chromosomes. We really felt that nothing could go wrong.

Until we found ourselves in beta hCG hell. My first blood test came back at 24, which was very low. We had to wait two days to measure it again. If it went up then the pregnancy might be ok, but if it went down, then we would lose the baby. I woke up very early that morning and took another pregnancy test. The pink line that I had seen earlier that week was gone. It was almost completely white. I crawled back into bed next to Jon and I knew I had to tell him.

"I'm so sorry Jon, I just took a test and I'm pretty sure that this pregnancy is over."

His silence said it all. We both lay there devastated, holding on tight to each other. Another blood test confirmed it, my hCG level was now 6. This was what is called a chemical pregnancy, meaning that the only way to confirm I was pregnant was by the chemicals in my blood. It was too early to see anything on an ultrasound.

How could this have happened? The embryo was perfect, it had passed pre-implantation testing, it was graded 6AB and it had implanted. We will never have any answers, because, like with many miscarriages, no one knows why. We have since found out that the chance of miscarriage in these circumstances is less that 5%. I guess we were just unlucky. We'll never know why that baby couldn't stay. The baby we were so excited about, that we had bonded with in such a short time.

I read a metaphor somewhere that PGS can tell you the number of pages in a book, it can't tell you what is written on the page. The embryo can have the correct number of chromosomes, but still have genetic problems. And it's not 100% accurate, it only checks a couple of pages from the book, it might not tell if there is a problem on some other pages. And sometimes embryos can self correct which might mean you could discard an embryo that would have worked. However, PGS testing is a wonderful tool if you have lots of embryos and need to figure out what order to transfer them in or if you have genetic issues or advanced maternal age or multiple losses. And it does reduce the chance of miscarriage, so you have to weigh up the cost, how many embryos you have and how much your heart can bear.

Maybe we were naïve, but we really believed that this pregnancy would continue. It was extremely painful to let go of our 'best' embryo, that we had thought about and prayed for the last 2 years. Part of me felt like it wasn't a 'real miscarriage' because it was so early. I have since come to understand that every pregnancy changes you, no matter how long it lasts. It might seem like a short time to some, but it was enough time to dream about that baby's entire life. A miscarriage is so much more than the loss of an embryo, it's the loss of a dream.

For us, there were even more implications. Now we only had 8 embryos left and only one of them was tested. Was there something else wrong with me or with my uterus that we had missed? We organised with our doctor to do the recurrent miscarriage blood panel, a hysteroscopy and a D and C surgery (dilation and curettage) to check if there was anything that could have made the environment unwelcoming to our precious, perfect embryo. We never got any answers.

We had nothing else to do but to try again and pray for a better outcome next time. We had to bolster our hearts and risk being hurt so badly yet again. We'll never forget you little AB, too perfect for this world.

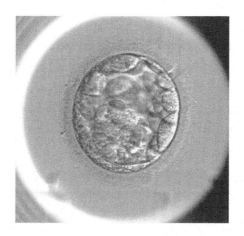

FROM JON

If you know what Laura and I have been though, I am certain the word 'naïve' doesn't come in to your mind. After seventeen runs around the IVF track, you would think we would have it all figured out. We have already done the hard yards, right? Unfortunately not. Even with our perfect embryo, our PGS tested embryo, her perfect uterus lining and the perfect implantation. Any reasonable person would think that was going to be a slam dunk. It was not.

I had so many feelings as we experienced the loss of this little soul. Feelings of guilt that I had put Laura through all of this stress. Blame. How did this go so wrong? I felt so sad and completely unprepared for this part of our journey. I honestly thought we had been lucky yet again. I felt frustrated that even though everything seemed perfect, it could still all go so, so wrong.

Our miscarriage was so emotionally painful, and no amount of positivity was going to keep me from feeling this one. I had to listen to Laura blaming herself and trying to seek answers that in all honesty, weren't there. All anyone could tell us was 'These things happen.' The pain of it stung in a way I had never felt before.

For me, 'resilience' is the word that comes up repeatedly as we go through infertility. The strength to take the hit, dust yourself off and forge forward using all that you have learned, however tough those lessons may be. I do not believe you can ever be prepared for your reaction to an experience like this, though if you attack these struggles with love, kindness and gratitude, you will make it through to the other side. I know deep down that together Laura and I can help each other through anything. Just look at what we have had to endure so far.

Goodbye little one, I will remember you always.

Thank you for gracing us with your presence, even if it was for just a fleeting moment.

You gave us so much, even though we didn't get to hold you in our arms. I will always love you and be your Dad.

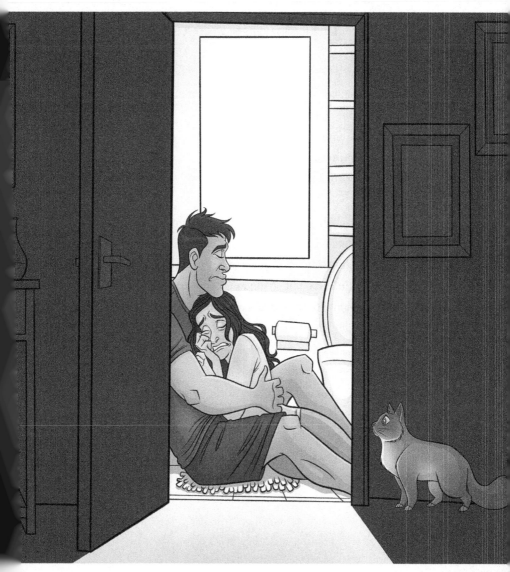

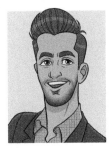

*When a man is unwell, I find they can often remain calm, stoic and strong, but when their partner is unwell, men really struggle. It's not unusual to see them crumble when their partner is not doing well. When a woman is miscarrying, it is a very tough time for the man. Whilst the physical burden of the miscarriage falls entirely on the woman, the emotional burden is shared. - **Dr Scott Shemer**

There are many points in a fertility journey where it is possible to experience loss:

▶ Learning that you have an infertility diagnosis. It may mean you cannot conceive naturally, carry a pregnancy or have a genetic connection to your child.

▶ A failed IVF cycle where no eggs or no embryos were produced.

▶ A failed sperm retrieval.

▶ Embryos, eggs or sperm that do not survive the freeze and thaw process.

▶ A failed transfer where an embryo was transferred, but it did not result in a pregnancy.

▶ A chemical pregnancy meaning you had a positive result on a pregnancy test, but it did not continue.

▶ An ectopic pregnancy, which occurs when the embryo implants somewhere outside the uterus, usually in the fallopian tube.

▶ A miscarriage, the loss of a pregnancy before 20 weeks, although this term can be used to describe all pregnancy loss.

▶ A stillbirth, losing a baby after 20 weeks of pregnancy.

▶ The donation of eggs, sperm or embryos that is cancelled.

▶ A surrogacy arrangement that falls through.

▶ An adoption that does not go ahead.

▶ Deciding that it is the end of one stage of a fertility journey.

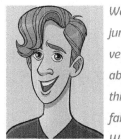

*We decided about three years ago that we were ready to jump in and add to our family. We actually fell pregnant very quickly but unfortunately we had a miscarriage at about the eight-week mark. It was pretty devastating. I think because we got pregnant easily, we were lulled into a false sense of security. It was quite a shock to the system. We tried again and we got pregnant again, pretty much straight away. Unfortunately, we had another miscarriage, this one didn't get quite as far along, it didn't make it past six weeks. That left us pretty shattered, as you can imagine. - **Carter**

Pregnancy Loss

Miscarriage is more common than most people think. It is estimated that 1 in 5 pregnancies end in miscarriage, with most of those losses occurring in the first 12 weeks. More than half of all first trimester miscarriages result from problems with the embryo's chromosomes. In most cases, the cause is something you couldn't have prevented, which means there is nothing that you or your partner could have done to prevent your miscarriage.

You did nothing wrong, and neither did she.

Some miscarriages can be dangerous to the woman's health, so it is important that you report whatever is happening to your doctor.

A miscarriage is complete when all the pregnancy tissue has passed. In very early miscarriage, this may just seem like a normal, or slightly heavier period. A miscarriage is called incomplete when some of the pregnancy tissue has passed, but some is still inside the uterus. A 'missed' miscarriage is when the pregnancy has stopped growing, but the tissue has not passed and there is still a sac (the structure surrounding the embryo or fetus) in the uterus.

Treatment of Miscarriage

Depending on when and how the miscarriage has occurred, you and your doctor will choose treatment options.

► Wait for the miscarriage to occur naturally, if it is safe to do so.

► Take medicine to assist her body to start bleeding.

► Undergo a dilation and curettage surgery (D and C) or a dilation and evacuation (D and E) to remove the fetus.

► An ectopic pregnancy will most likely require surgery and possibly the removal of the fallopian tubes.

► For miscarriages in later stages of pregnancy, a pregnant person may go into labour or have a caesarean delivery.

Seek some answers

Most of the time, patients will never know the cause of their miscarriage. However, there are some tests which can be undertaken at the time of the miscarriage and afterwards which might give you some answers.

It may be possible to test the tissue from the miscarried fetus to see if there were any genetic issues. Many people learn through this testing that their embryo was never capable of growing and surviving which can bring some peace and further confirm that the miscarriage was not their fault.

After experiencing a miscarriage, talk to your doctor about any additional tests that may help to explain what happened and prevent it from happening again. Some women may have structural abnormalities in their uterus, which can be treated if identified. There may be extra blood tests she can have to check for autoimmune, genetic, thyroid or blood clotting factors that may shed some light on how to prevent miscarriages in the future.

Emotional Effects

People who have experienced loss may have a range of feelings. There are no right or wrong emotions to feel at this time, and everyone is different. Some common emotions that you or your partner might feel after a reproductive loss are shock, numbness, anxiety, disbelief, denial, sadness, guilt, anger, envy, distraction, despair, loneliness, depression and concern about the future.

Every reproductive loss is different. Sometimes the amount of upset is not comparable to what might be perceived as the size of the loss. This is really important to remember when interacting with your partner, as she might feel some losses more than others, regardless of how she 'should' feel based on the level of loss.

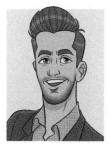

A patient of mine had a diagnosed missed miscarriage at about 10 weeks. She was really upset. Her husband kept saying, 'Don't worry about it, it's fine, it's all going to be ok, we'll be alright.' That was not what she wanted to hear in that moment. I didn't want him to feel bad about the fact that he was trying to be positive but at the same time I wanted to say 'I think it's really wonderful that you are trying to stay positive and you're focussing on the future, but this is a really hard thing to go through and you need to allow yourselves time to grieve.' Positivity and looking to the future does have a place, but in the moment of loss, the focus should be on experiencing it and giving the appropriate time and space for it to be processed. - Dr Scott Shemer

Your age, length of gestation, history of previous pregnancy and IVF losses, the amount of money and time devoted to conceiving are all important factors that can affect the intensity of emotional pain.

- ▶ Is it the last chance or the first try?
- ▶ Did you expect it to work, or did you have realistic expectations that it might not work?
- ▶ Did you spend a lot of money on fertility treatment (in relation to your financial situation)?
- ▶ Did the pregnancy last for a short time or a long time?
- ▶ Is the woman considered old or young in fertility terms?
- ▶ How much fertility treatment have you already been through?
- ▶ Will you be able to get pregnant again easily or not?
- ▶ Do you have children already or not?
- ▶ Are things happening around you that make you more vulnerable at this time (such as your best friend having a baby)?

The answers to these questions may help to understand why a person is grieving, but regardless of the answers, every person has the right to feel grief for any reason at any time.

There are also some apparently unrelated factors that can intensify reproductive grief, such as the early loss of your own parents, a history of sexual abuse or simply the story we have in our head of how our fertility journey should play out.

In the end, any kind of loss can have a significant emotional impact, and it doesn't matter what has happened, what really matters is how we feel about it. So when taking care of yourself and your partner, be gentle and allow yourselves to feel whatever emotions show up and don't judge how you feel or compare yourselves to others.

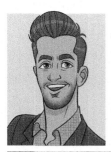

The partner will often try to be stoic and supportive for the person going through the pregnancy loss. There is nothing he can do to salvage the pregnancy, but he can be there to support the woman through what is probably one of the worst experiences of her life. And it is important to recognise that it is a tough time for him as well. **- Dr Scott Shemer**

It's not so simple to just 'get over' a reproductive loss. It changes who you are, but you can learn to live with it. Over time, you will find a way to accept it and perhaps even draw some strength or beauty from the experience. As devastating as it is, eventually time will allow you to rebuild and things will ultimately improve.

Some people will fixate on time in relation to the pregnancy. For example, they will pay attention to what point they would have been in the pregnancy, had it continued to a live birth. She might visit pregnancy websites and obsess over symptoms she would have had at 28 weeks, 29 weeks and so on. The baby's due date may be an especially difficult day. Even after the due date, thoughts of how old the baby would have been, or how they might have looked, can preoccupy your mind. To make it worse, others around you or your partner might not understand this need to track the lost baby's progress, making you or her feel even more misunderstood.

Sometimes these emotions can be misdirected and you may feel angry with others, such as your partner, your boss or the medical staff. You might fixate on a particular comment or feeling that if the doctors had acknowledged your concerns differently, then maybe the outcome would have been different. Try to remember that this misdirected anger is not necessarily helpful and can sometimes act as a way for you to avoid the way you are really feeling, which is sadness at the failure of your treatment or the loss of your pregnancy.

You and your partner may experience disruption in your life, such as:

► fatigue

► sleep disturbance (difficulty sleeping or sleeping too much)

► appetite disturbance (loss of appetite or overeating)

► inability to concentrate

► breathing difficulties

► anxiety

► tension

► irritability

Depending on your situation, be aware your partner may be experiencing physical symptoms at the same time as the emotional impact.

► If she was taking fertility medications, her hormone levels may be out of whack.

► If she experienced miscarriage, not only will her hormones be changing back to normal, but she may also be experiencing bleeding, cramping and possible infection.

► If she had an incomplete miscarriage, she may need surgical intervention.

► If she was further along in the pregnancy, she may have to go through labour or she might even be producing breast milk, which is an incredibly upsetting reminder of what you have lost.

These physical symptoms might make it even more challenging for her to process the emotions she is experiencing. She will rely on you to be her rock and at the same time, it's very important that you take care of yourself because you have also experienced a difficult loss.

Family and Friends

Many people do not announce their pregnancy or tell people they are undergoing fertility treatment. This can cause an internal struggle when a loss is experienced. Should you tell friends and family now?

People experiencing reproductive loss can feel a profound sense of loneliness as it feels like no one understands what this experience is like.

Throughout history, people were expected to grieve pregnancy loss in private. Thankfully, this is no longer the case. If it makes sense for you to share your grief, then do so. It is wonderful to see so many couples sharing their experiences as this hopefully helps them to process their own grief, but also lets others know they are not alone.

There are virtually no rituals or cultural norms for grieving a miscarriage or infertility. So come up with some of your own if you decide this will help. It might be appropriate to hold some kind of ceremony to commemorate the lost child. You might just like to write something, make something or buy something as a way of remembering them. You might also like to commemorate a lost embryo, perhaps with a journal entry, choosing a name or with a special gift such as a piece of jewellery.

Remembering and acknowledging the child, pregnancy or fertility experience can be an important part of the grieving process. However, you need to be sure that this is working for you and not against you. If remembering the loss is taking up a lot of time or interfering with other parts of your life, then you may need to seek help to learn to reduce those activities and focus more on living your life beyond your loss.

After a certain amount of time, you will need to resume some of your regular activities. You'll go back to work, have to cook and clean and pay your bills. This can be a difficult time as it can sometimes hurt even more to see how the world has continued as normal, when your entire world has come crashing down around you. The loss of a pregnancy or failed fertility treatment is an experience that will remain with you throughout your life. We're not saying this to be negative, it is simply the truth, and to reassure you that you are not expected to 'just get over it'. Rest assured, with time you will figure out how to live a happy life, with reproductive loss as a part of your story.

So, What Can We Do?

How can you, as a man, experience your own emotions through this loss? And how can you support your partner as she goes through it with you?

- ► Be open to asking for help. Reaching out for support is the bravest thing you can ever do.
- ► Talk to friends, family or a professional about how you are feeling.
- ► Take care of your physical health. A healthy diet, exercise and sleep help when you are going through challenging times.
- ► Do things you enjoy even if you don't really feel like it.
- ► Be aware of your stress levels. Reduce your workload as much as you can, actively relax through meditation, music, or anything else that makes you feel good. And you deserve to feel good.

How to help yourself or someone else experiencing grief and loss

Although it may feel difficult during this time, make sure that you and your partner are taking care of yourselves through the grieving process. Do your best to continue routines in your daily life.

Here are some practical things you can do that can really help both you and your partner:

- ► Drink plenty of water.
- ► Make sure you have bathed and put on clean clothes.
- ► Eat several healthy meals a day
- ► Keep the house tidy.
- ► Set up a good sleep routine in a comfortable environment. Make sure the room is dark and the bed sheets are clean and fresh.
- ► Maintain appropriate caffeine and alcohol intake. Avoid drugs or prescription medication misuse.
- ► Participate in gentle exercise, such as a walk in the park or yoga.

- Meditate.
- Keep in touch with family and friends and let them know how to help. Keep interactions with visitors brief and positive.
- Do an activity that you enjoy.
- Take a break from thinking about your loss, whatever that means to you.
- Play soothing music or nature sounds.
- Light a scented candle or use an essential oil diffuser.
- Engage in pleasurable activities and activities that make you feel a sense of accomplishment.

If your partner is struggling with grief, you may be able to take some simple steps to help her get through:

- Ask how she is feeling. Each day can be different, so take the time to listen and understand. You don't need to provide solutions, just listening and being present with her is the best thing you can do. Turn your phone off during these conversations.
- Ask her how you can help. This might be doing extra around the house to reduce her stress, going for a walk or watching a funny movie with her. She may not be able to articulate what will help her, so be patient and gently offer suggestions.
- Assist her with remembering any medications she needs to take or doctor's appointments she needs to attend. Set alarms and reminders.
- When appropriate, help to distract her from thinking about the loss, for example, encourage a hobby or craft activity that she enjoys.
- Make her a cup of tea.
- Give her a gentle massage.
- In really difficult moments, connect and help her breathe deeply.
- Talk about everyday life too. The loss you have experienced doesn't need to be at the centre of every conversation.
- Most of all, give her lots of big hugs.

When to get help

Speak to a counsellor or therapist if you feel it may help, especially if the grief does not seem to be easing. Seek professional support if you or your partner:

▶ are having regular or intrusive flashbacks or nightmares about the experience of your loss.

▶ are experiencing emotions that interfere with your ability to work or basically take care of yourself or others for whom you are responsible.

▶ are engaging in self-destructive acts, such as harming yourself, excessive alcohol or drug use, promiscuity or spending money beyond your means.

▶ are experiencing suicidal thoughts.

It might be useful to look for a therapist that has experience working with infertility, miscarriage and reproductive loss. Sometimes that can be found through your fertility clinic or your general doctor. There are also specific help groups, online groups and treatment centres that are devoted to pregnancy loss.

You and your partner will take the path to healing that is right for you. It might take some time, but you will begin to feel more like yourself. This loss will always be a part of your story, but compassion for each other and self-care will help you move through your grief and look forward to feeling happier once again.

FROM LAURA

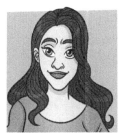

Some of the strongest and bravest people I know are part of my circle of infertility warriors. They fight the stereotypes of infertility, and they advocate tirelessly for themselves with friends, family, and healthcare professionals. They are relentlessly resilient and hopeful. Get to know some real men and women who have been through multiple rounds of IVF. There's nothing weak or broken about them.

THE AFTERMATH OF INFERTILITY

LEFTOVER EGGS, SPERM AND EMBRYOS

When you are no longer pursuing fertility treatment or you feel that you have completed your family, there are sometimes some frosty little leftovers. What do you do with frozen embryos, eggs or sperm?

People who have frozen embryos they are not intending to use often find it hard to decide what to do. If you have some little ones in the freezer, you will need to pay a storage fee for them annually. It's not unusual for people who have completed their families to pay the fee every year, unsure of how to progress. It is difficult to let go of something that was so difficult to create and that holds so much potential. It is challenging to decide what to do with them.

Here are your options:
1. Use them to try for another baby.
2. Discard them.
3. Donate them to another family.
4. Donate them for research.

As always, only you can know what is the best choice for you. Take your time to make the decision; there is really no rush. Compared to the amount you paid for IVF the storage fee is quite small. However, don't push it out of your mind for too long. Every time that storage invoice arrives, take some time to actively think about your options and sit down to speak with your partner. Do some research about what would happen if you donated them. If you feel confident with one of the options, bravely take that step. If not, pay the invoice and revisit it again next time, just make sure that you are taking the time to think through your options.

PREGNANCY AFTER INFERTILITY

Hopefully, at some point you will be able to celebrate the end of the chapter of your life called 'Infertility' with the start of a new chapter called 'Pregnancy'. Congratulations!

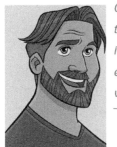

*Our 6th cycle, we had a mega haul of 26 eggs, 19 of them were mature and fertilised, but only one made it over the line. That one became our baby. Once the embryo took, we had a really uncomplicated pregnancy, which was fantastic for our anxiety levels! - **Josh***

It should be all smooth sailing from here, right? Not so fast. The transition from infertile to pregnant can be so sudden that it can send you into shock. Your partner may go from IVF medications and egg pick ups directly to morning sickness. It can be quite a whirlwind. Emotionally, it can take a while for your identity to shift from 'infertile' to 'newly pregnant'. The way other people treat you can shift dramatically too.

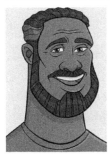

*After going through so much to have him, our first feeling when our baby was finally conceived was not joy, but disbelief. It was surreal; I don't think either of us could accept it had actually happened and was going to last. We'd had so many ups and downs that we couldn't believe that nothing bad was going to happen. - **Michael***

Feeling Anxious

It can sometimes take a while for you and your partner to process being pregnant. Becoming pregnant after infertility or reproductive loss can bring with it a lot of fear and apprehension. Most pregnant women feel a little anxious - that is a normal part of pregnancy. This anxiety can increase dramatically when she has experienced difficulty conceiving or a previous loss or trauma. It can be a stressful time if you have spent loads of cash and energy in getting pregnant in the first place.

After being in all those online chat groups where members post about failed IVF cycles, miscarriages and stillbirths, women often have a heightened awareness of what can go wrong during pregnancy.

About 20% of pregnancies end in miscarriage and once a pregnancy is confirmed, the rate for IVF pregnancies is about the same. You will likely both feel better once you can feel your baby kicking, which happens sometime between 16 and 25 weeks. For many, the anxiety doesn't really go away until the baby is born, when it will be replaced by the normal concerns that come with parenting. Celebrate every week that goes by with your partner and remind her that every week is a step closer to holding your baby in your arms.

But I'm Supposed To Be Happy!

Pregnancy is pretty uncomfortable for most women. When a woman has been through infertility, she may be reluctant to express any negative feelings during pregnancy because she feels she should be grateful to be pregnant at all. However, mixed feelings during pregnancy are normal.

▶ Let her know it is ok to say how she is really feeling even if it is negative.
▶ Explain to her you know she is still grateful for the pregnancy.
▶ Tell her you are excited to experience all of the pregnancy with her including her complaining about morning sickness or sore feet!

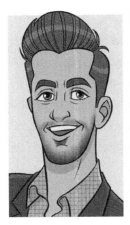

Medical Care

Pregnancy after infertility can be quite triggering. Having been through IVF myself, my patients really know that I understand. Getting through a pregnancy isn't just about getting optimal medical care; it's also about getting the emotional support that can help you enjoy the pregnancy. This extra support goes beyond my role as a doctor, it is just about being a compassionate human being. All pregnancies are incredibly precious. Personally, I don't consider my non-IVF child any less precious than my IVF child. All babies are miraculous and wonderful however as an obstetrician, I do treat pregnancies after infertility differently.

- *Firstly, the patient might require different care because of a medical or physical indication. The same factors that have contributed to their infertility may also impact on the pregnancy. For example, some women might need IVF because they're older or very obese and therefore they are already at higher risk of miscarriage, fetal abnormality or other complications. So, I want to see them more often than other patients in the first trimester because they may be more likely to have complications.*

- *Secondly, I offer additional reassurance and support to all families who have been through fertility treatment for emotional reasons. I see them more often in the first trimester, usually at weekly appointments. There is anxiety that comes with having taken so long to fall pregnant, or because they have used IVF for genetic conditions or they have suffered previous pregnancy losses. These are families that are used to receiving sub-optimal news, and that is why they have that heightened level of anxiety.*

Top Tip

If a patient has gotten pregnant easily and they come in for their first appointment, I will book in all of their subsequent appointments and discuss the whole pregnancy, right up to the birth. For people who have been through a difficult fertility journey, I find that taking smaller steps can be a better strategy.

Rather than sitting down at the first appointment and talking about what we're going to do at 39 and 40 weeks, I say to them, 'Why don't we just talk about what is going to happen in the next 2 to 3 weeks? Why don't we break this down into smaller time periods and focus on them one at a time, so that we're not getting too far ahead of ourselves?'

I do this not because I'm concerned about the pregnancy or being pessimistic but because I feel this can be a better way to manage the anxiety that can come with pregnancy after infertility. Once we get through the first trimester, then we will talk in much more detail about what lies ahead.

- Dr Scott Shemer

Stepping Away From Infertility

It's a good idea to think about your shifting identity as you embark on your new adventure. You may have to take active steps to help you and your partner transition.

► Journal and write about your emotions. This can help you make the shift.

► Consider if it might feel good to remove yourself from online infertility support groups. This can be helpful to you, and it is also kind to the people who are still trying to conceive and may find it difficult to discuss your pregnancy.

► Put away any IVF medications or other items around the house that remind you of infertility.

► Make a gradual transition from fertility treatment into regular pregnancy care by choosing an obstetrician or midwife program.

► Send a thank you card to your fertility clinic to help you close that chapter of your life.

► Purchase something for the baby; this can help it to feel more real.

► Tell a few of your close friends and family. You may not feel ready to share the news with the entire world, but sharing with a few people could help you feel the excitement and provide you with support.

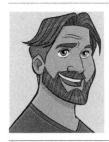

*I'm a very sensitive human, I tear up watching a cat food commercial. But during my journey through IVF I didn't shed a single tear... until my daughter was born and then I f***ing lost it. When we were a couple of days before the birth I was in the fetal position, just bawling. It was really good to finally have that release. - **Josh***

Consider Counselling

You may want to seek some professional help to process your experience of infertility. It might be a good idea to do that before the baby comes. Some couples experience a kind of post-traumatic stress after having a difficult time trying to conceive. Many don't feel like they are allowed to talk about it, because they think they are supposed to be immediately joyful in their pregnancy. This time should be whatever it needs to be, in order for you to move forward in the best way possible for you, your partner, and your baby.

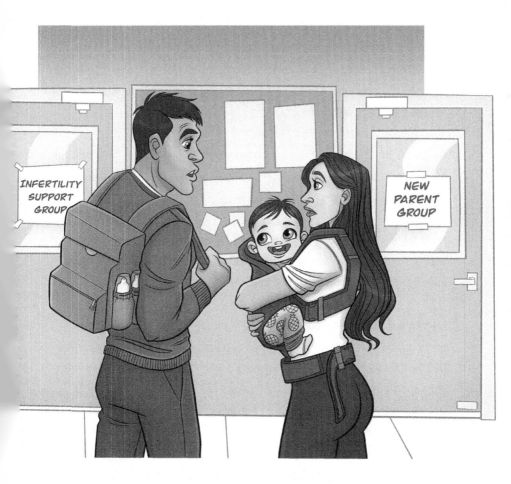

FROM LAURA

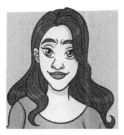

It took me a long time to feel comfortable with the idea that I was pregnant. We didn't tell anyone about the baby until I was 13 weeks along and even then only close family and friends. It just didn't seem real. I felt pretty guilty that I had been so lucky. I had come to know and care for other women who were going through infertility, either through my clinic or online. Why had I been so lucky when they had not?

Physically, I was pretty run down. I had done 15 cycles of IVF egg retrievals, many of them back-to-back. Suddenly I experienced an onslaught of new and different pregnancy symptoms, when I only just felt like I was recovering from the IVF symptoms. My hormones were only starting to rebalance after fertility treatment, when the pregnancy hormones set in.

I was definitely happy, but I also felt other conflicting emotions. I was anxious about the pregnancy, nervous about telling people and even feeling guilty about the fact that I was happy.

I had spent so much energy over a 3-year period avoiding anything to do with pregnancy. Being around pregnant women usually made me feel sad or uncomfortable, but now I was one of them. How do you reconcile that?

I remember sitting in my obstetrician's office before an appointment. On every other chair in the waiting room was a pregnant woman. I started to feel that familiar sense of dread washing over me, hoping that they wouldn't start chatting about pregnancy. I had been in uncomfortable situations before, pretending to be happy about others' pregnancies while feeling so sad for myself. I dropped my eyes to avoid eye contact, only to see that my own belly was round and pregnant. It felt like I was in some kind of dream. It took me a long time to truly believe that I had a baby on the way.

MOVING FORWARD WITHOUT CHILDREN

FROM JON

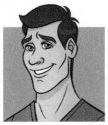 *This was the hardest part of this book to write.*
Who are we to tell you how to manage the experience
of choosing to remain childless?
Your situation and your emotions are unique to you.
No one will ever truly understand what this has been
like for you, because your experience is one of a kind. No one can truly
understand the years that it has taken you and your partner to get to this
point. Except maybe people who have had to make similar decisions.
We can certainly empathise and send you love. We hope you get support
that will help you feel empowered by your decisions.

Living without children after infertility is an option some men and women choose, and some must come to accept. Initially, you may have seen living child free as the worst-case scenario. However, for many people who have gone down this path, it can be an empowering resolution to an emotionally exhausting situation.

Some feel the term 'child free' doesn't reflect the emotional pain they went through to reach this place in their life. It more accurately describes those who actually chose to be without children from the beginning. 'Childless not by choice' or 'childless by chance' is perhaps a more accurate term for those who wanted children but could not have them.

Many feel that the term 'childless' is too negative, that it doesn't accurately describe the joyful life they are now living, even if living without children wasn't their Plan A. In the end the words you use to describe your life are up to you.

There is a certain peace to envisioning a life not driven by menstrual cycles and heartbreaking waiting periods. After exhaustive conversations with your partner, it can bring relief to loosen your tight grip on a fragile dream.

You might find yourself considering this option when you are tired of living in limbo, when the heartbreak of IVF failures and pregnancy losses is too much to bear – especially when most of the world didn't recognise your losses or offer the kinds of support reserved for other types of grief. After so many years of living through infertility, with so many things outside of your control, you can finally start to see your life as your own, where you can make choices and be more confident in the outcomes.

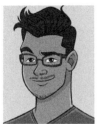 *Finally deciding that you won't have kids is a tough decision. And it's not always entirely your decision, is it? There is a lot you can't control. There are a lot of people who have chased after hope and they've run after unicorns and spent thousands and thousands of dollars trying to have a baby. Sometimes you just don't end up with the result you're hoping for. You end up with a broken heart, an empty bank account, and maybe even a broken relationship. Kids are great, but you can also have an amazing life without them. So think clearly and calmly about what steps you take. Because there is a great life to be had, whatever you decide to do. - Brett*

Navigating the emotional journey towards being happy in a life without children is an ongoing process. Once people have grieved and made a definite decision to remain child free, they tend to feel occasional twinges of sadness, but no more stabbing pain when they consider the life for which they had previously hoped.

If you need to be sad about it, that's fine but if being sad about it doesn't change it, you need to be really clear about how long you want to be sad. There's too much life to live to suffer over something that you can't change.

No one else can decide for you whether living without children is right for you. Deciding not to have a child does not take away the meaning of those years of trying. It's your life. You have the right to decide what to do with it.

FROM JON

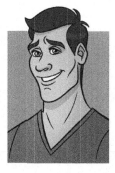

For 10 years, I believed I was infertile and that I would never have children. During that time, I decided to get involved in the lives of other people's kids, hoping that I could be a positive influence before handing them back to their parents. I found my particular calling in mentoring teenagers, who have a great need for empowering leadership. I am very grateful for those years when I truly believed I would remain childless, because they opened up in me a new calling to become a better man and impact the world in ways other than parenting.

SHARE YOUR STORY

Once you have reached the end of your fertility journey, you will not be the same person you were at the beginning. You will have experienced some very challenging times and learnt so much along the way.

Somehow, the people at the start of their journey will find you. Share what you now know, you will help them in a way that only one who has been through it can.

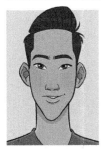

If sharing our story can help even just one couple, that makes it worth it. The stories of others helped us. The people willing to share their stories, their tears, their happiness, their fears, all of it. Even the successes, which we know that can be a little sensitive because there are people who still don't have their dream yet. They might not be in a place yet where they can hear all the happy stories. We really want to give back because hearing from the community really helped us. - James

CONCLUSION

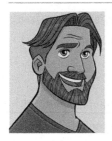

Looking back, I wouldn't have done anything differently. It's very easy to have 'what-ifs.' We inevitably made mistakes you don't even really want to think about. All I can really say is that we made the best decisions we could with the information we had at the time. We couldn't have done anything differently. - Josh

When infertility touches your life, it makes an indelible mark. Infertility changes your perspective. You will develop a compassion for the things people go through behind closed doors and an extra appreciation for any roles you get to play in children's lives.

Though it will make its mark on your life, your infertility journey won't last forever. You will move through the stages and the mindsets and you will come out the other side. We'll be supporting you the whole way.

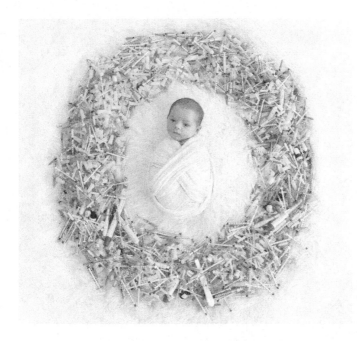

FROM JON AND LAURA

Feel free to get in touch with us online through www.InfertilityMan.com. We'd love to hear about your experiences and how you have overcome your challenges.

We hope you'll find ways to grow and to be happy, strong and fulfilled while going through infertility and on the other side. Thank you for sharing some of our stories. We wish you the very best in yours.

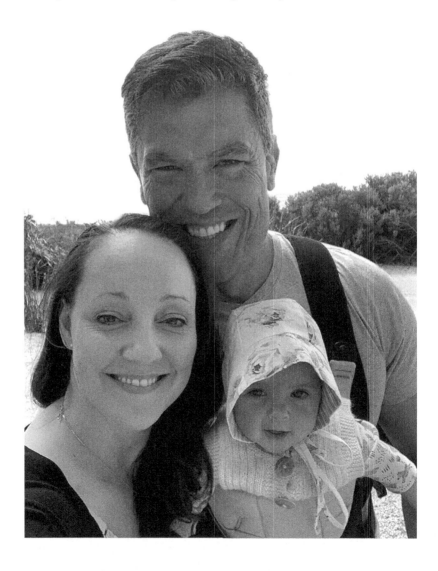

Leave Us a Review

We hope you enjoyed this book. We poured our hearts into it and included everything we learned while trying to conceive our own kids. We hope it helps people going through similar experiences. We're just a normal couple who faced difficulties with having children, as so many families do. Infertility is such a challenging journey, and we were so grateful to all those who helped us, so we wrote this book to pay it forward to the next group of people who need support.

Please consider sharing a book review. We really want to reach as many people as possible and that is how you can help us. If you can write a few sentences, film a video talking about the book or share a photo of yourself with the book on social media, it would be an enormous help.

Make sure you tag us or write to us to let us know about your review, we'd love to meet you and thank you personally.

Reviews make it easier for more people to find this book, which will hopefully make them feel more connected and supported as they try to conceive or build their own families.

www.InfertilityMan.com/Reviews

GLOSSARY

2WW	Two-Week Wait - The waiting period between ovulation or embryo transfer and a pregnancy test.
AC	Assisted Conception - Medical help to concieve a baby
AF	Aunt Flo - Period or Menstrual Cycle.
AFC	Antral Follicle Count - Indicator of ovarian reserve – often at the start of the cycle. The number of follicles present in the ovary.
AMA	Advanced Maternal Age - The age of the female, indicating she is near the end of her reproductive years.
AMH	Anti-Mullerian Hormone - Hormone levels used to assess egg reserve.
Aneuploidy	Aneuploidy - Abnormal number of chromosomes in a cell.
AO	Anovulatory - The lack or absence of ovulation.
ART	Assisted Reproductive Technology - Fertility treatments.
ASA	Antisperm Antibody - Damages sperm and is found in blood and vaginal fluid.
Asthenozoospermia	Sperm Condition - Reduced sperm motility in the ejaculate.
BBT	Basal Body Temperature - Your temperature when fully at rest, used to track the cycle of ovulation.
BCP	Birth Control Pills - Contraception.
BD	Baby Dance - Sex with the intention of conceiving.
Beta	HcG Pregnancy Test - Human chorionic gonadotropin levels in the blood or urine to assesses for pregnancy.
BFN	Big Fat Negative - Negative pregnancy test.
BFP	Big Fat Positive - Positive pregnancy test.
Blastocyst	Embryo - At 5–7 days development with a complex cellular structure.
BMI	Body Mass Index - Measurement tool using height to weight range.
BMS	Baby-Making Sex - Sex with the intention of conceiving.
BW	Blood Work - Pathology.
C#	Cycle Number - Indicates how many cycles of fertility treatment have been undertaken.
CB	Cycle Buddy - Another person going through fertility treatment at the same time.
CD	Cycle Day - A day of the menstrual cycle.
CGH	Comparative Genomic Hybridisation A DNA diagnostic technique to check for chromosomal abnormalities.
Clomid	Clomiphene; Chloramifene; Chloramiphene; Fertility medication used to jumpstart ovulation.
CM	Cervical Mucus/Fluid - The cervix produces this due to increased oestrogen as ovulation approaches.
CoQ10	Co-Enzyme Q10/Ubiquinol - Naturally produced antioxidant for the growth and maintenance of cells. Can be taken in pill or oil form.
CP	Cervical Position - Position of the cervix.
CS	Caesarean Section - A surgical operation for delivering a child by cutting through the wall of the woman's abdomen.
CVS	Chorionic Villi Sampling - A test for genetic abnormalities during pregnancy i.e. Downs syndrome.
DD	Dear Daughter
DE	Donor Eggs - Oocytes donated to allow another woman to become pregnant.
DH	Dear Husband

DHEA	Dehydroepiandrosterone - A hormone naturally produced in the adrenal gland, it helps produce other hormones, including testosterone and oestrogen. Can be taken in pill or oil form.
DOR	Diminished Ovarian Reserve - A condition that compromises fertility where the ovary loses its normal reproductive potential.
DP	Dear Partner
DPO	Days Post Ovulation
DPR	Days Post Retrieval
DPT	Days Post Transfer
DS	Dear Son
DS	Donor Sperm - Sperm donated to fertilise an egg and enable a woman to become pregnant.
DW	Dear Wife
Dx	Diagnosis - Identifying the nature of the medical problem/challenge.
E2	Oestrogen - This hormone promotes follicle growth.
ED	Egg Donor - A person who donates their eggs for someone else to use.
Ejaculation	Post Orgasm - Discharge of semen containing sperm.
EDD	Estimated Due Date - Approximate date when the delivery of a baby is expected.
Endo	Endometriosis - Tissue similar to the uterine internal lining grows outside the uterus.
Endometrium	The lining of the uterus.
Epididymis	Male Reproductive Part - Part of the testes that stores sperm prior to ejaculation.
EPO	Evening Primrose Oil - A rich source of omega-6 essential fatty acids. May be taken orally.
EPT	Early Pregnancy Test - A more sensitive type of urine test.
EPU	Egg Pick-Up - Surgical procedure to collect eggs from the ovaries (OPU also).
ER	Egg Retrieval - Surgical procedure to collect eggs from the ovaries (OPU also).
ET	Embryo Transfer - Insertion of the embryo into the uterus.
EWCM	Egg White Cervical Mucus Fertile cervical mucus, with the consistency of egg whites.
FA/FzAll	Freeze All - All eggs or embryos created are frozen.
Fallopian Tubes	Female Reproductive Part - Tubes joining the ovaries and the uterus for transport of oocyte; usually the site of fertilisation.
FERT	Fertilisation - Oocytes fertilised.
Fertilisation	Egg and sperm combine to form an embryo.
FET	Frozen Embryo Transfer - Frozen eggs used for transfer.
Fresh Embryo Transfer	An embryo that has not previously been frozen is used for transfer.
FF	Female Factor - Fertility challenges caused by diagnosis in the female.
FHR	Foetal Heart Rate - Heart rate of an unborn foetus.
FMU	First Morning Urine - Collected from the first urination of the day.
FNA	Fine Needle Aspiration - A blind sperm retrieval technique using a needle inserted into the testicle.
Follicle	Found in the ovaries, may contain an Oocyte (Egg) the uterus.
FP	Follicular Phase - The part of the menstrual cycle just before ovulation,
Fragmentation	Cells - Cell division error resulting in small pieces being excluded.
FRER	First Response Early Result - Early pregnancy test.
Frostie	Frozen Embryo - Embryo frozen for future use.

FS	Frozen Sperm - Sperm frozen for future use.
FS	Fertility Specialist - A doctor specialising in fertility treatment.
FSH (Women)	Follicle-Stimulating Hormone (Women) - In women this hormone helps control the menstrual cycle and egg production by the ovaries.
FSH (Men)	Follicle-Stimulating Hormone (Men) - In men this hormone stimulates testicular growth and enhances the production of an androgen-binding protein by the Sertoli cells, which are a component of the testicular tubule necessary for sustaining the maturing sperm cell.
FTF	Failed To Fertilise - Failure of oocytes & sperm to achieve fertilisation.
FTT	Failure To Thaw - Failure of frozen embryos, eggs or sperm to recover from the freezing and thawing process.
FTTA	Fertile Thoughts To All - A good luck wish.
GIFT	Gamete Intrafallopian Transfer - Eggs and sperm retrieved and inserted into the fallopian tubes to fertilise.
GnRH	Gonadotropin Releasing Hormone - A hormone that triggers the release of FSH.
HALO testing	Laboratory Test - Test on semen for damage and DNA fragmentation to sperm cells.
HcG	Human Chorionic Gonadotropin - The hormone detected by pregnancy tests
HGH	Human Growth Hormone - Naturally produced hormone by the body and can be supplemented.
HPT	Home Pregnancy Test - Pregnancy test at home.
HSG	Hysterosalpingogram - A test where fluid is run through the fallopian tubes to check for blockages.
IBT	Immunobead Testing - Semen test checking for antibodies that affect the sperm's ability to swim.
IC	Incompetent Cervix - When weak cervical tissue causes or contributes to premature birth or the loss of an otherwise healthy pregnancy.
IC	Intercourse - Sexual activity.
ICSI	Intracytoplasmic Sperm Injection Insemination of an egg with one sperm which is microinjected.
IF	Infertility - The inability to reproduce naturally.
IM	Intra Muscular Injection
IMSI	Intracytoplasmic Morphologically Selected Sperm Injection - An extra level of sperm selection using a more powerful microscope to exclude suspected abnormalities.
IR	Insulin Resistant - A resistance to the hormone insulin, resulting in increasing blood sugar.
IUI	Intrauterine Insemination - Sperm is washed and deposited in the uterus via the cervix.
IV	Intravenous - Giving medicines or fluids through a needle or tube inserted into a vein.
IVF	In Vitro Fertilisation - Eggs collected and inseminated with sperm to achieve fertilisation.
LAP	Laparoscopy - A type of diagnostic surgical procedure to look inside the abdomen at the reproductive organs. The surgeon can remove endometriosis scarring and lesions during the laparoscopy.
LH (Women)	Luteinizing Hormone - Hormone that triggers ovulation in females.
LH (Men)	Luteinizing Hormone - Hormone that stimulates the production of testosterone from Leydig cells in the testes in males.
LMP	Last Menstrual Period (Start Date) - Pregnancies are usually dated in weeks starting from the first day of a woman's last menstrual period.
LO	Little One - A baby or child.
LO	Left Ovary
LSC	Low Sperm Count - Low amount of sperm in the ejaculate.

MAI	Miscarriage After Infertility - Spontaneous loss of a pregnancy after infertility.
MC, m/c, misc.	Miscarriage - Spontaneous loss of a pregnancy.
MESA	Microsurgical Epididymal Sperm Aspiration - Sperm retrieval technique directly from the tubule when a blockage cannot be rectified.
Metformin	Diabetes Medication - A diabetes medication to assist in managing insulin and blood sugar levels in women with PCOS.
MF	Male Factor - Fertility challenges caused by diagnosis in the male.
Morphology	Characteristic - Shape characteristic of sperm cells.
MT	MicroTESE (Microscopic Testicular Sperm Extraction) - Using a microscope during surgery to select the most active tubules.
Multinucleate	Cells - Cells that have more than one nucleus per cell & can have more than one sperm enter and activate inside the oocyte.
NT	Nuchal Translucency Scan - A test for chromosomal abnormalities during pregnancy.
NIPT	Non-Invasive Prenatal Testing - A DNA-based blood test that screens for common genetic conditions in the developing foetus.
O,OV	Ovulation - A process where the egg is released from the ovaries.
OB	Open Biopsy - Removal of testicular tissue directly from the testis through a surgical opening.
OB, OB/GYN	Obstetrician/Gynaecologist - Specialist doctor for pregnancy and women's health.
OC	Oral Contraceptives - Oral birth control medications.
OHSS	Ovarian Hyperstimulation Syndrome - An exaggerated response to hormones in fertility medications. Worst symptoms can include severe abdominal pain, severe nausea or vomiting, decreased urination, dark-coloured urine, shortness of breath, low blood pressure and excessive weight gain.
OI	Ovulation Induction - A fertility treatment that induces ovulation.
Oligozoospermia	Sperm Condition - A reduced sperm count in the ejaculate.
OPK/OPT	Ovulation Predictor Kit, Ovulation Predictor Test - Urine test that measures the LH surge that precedes ovulation.
OPU	Oocyte Pick-Up - Surgical procedure. Egg collection from the ovaries.
OT	Ovulation Tracking - Tracking the menstrual cycle through blood tests & ultrasounds.
OTC	Over The Counter - Medications able to be purchased without prescription.
OV	Oocyte Vitrification - Snap freezing eggs.
Ovary/Ovaries	Female Reproductive Part - The female reproductive tissues / gonads.
OW	Oocyte Warming - Thawing eggs.
P4	Progesterone - Hormone involved in the menstrual cycle, pregnancy, and embryogenesis of humans and other species. Released by the corpus luteum in the ovary post ovulation. Can be taken as a medication.
PCOS	Polycystic Ovaries, Polycystic Ovarian Syndrome - A hormonal disorder causing enlarged ovaries with small cysts on the outer edges. Symptoms include menstrual irregularity, excess hair growth, acne and obesity.
PESA	Percutaneous Epididymal Sperm Aspiration - A sperm extraction technique when there is a blockage.
Pessary	Hormone Release Method - A prosthetic device or gel capsule inserted into the vagina for structural and pharmaceutical purposes, often used to deliver progesterone.
PG	Pregnant - Fertilisation has occurred and a foetus is developing inside the uterus.
PGD/PGS	Pre-Implantation Genetic Diagnosis/Pre-Implantation Genetic Screening - Testing of embryos for chromosomal defects prior to transfer.
PI	Primary Infertility - Refers to people who have no previous children and are having difficulty conceiving.
PICSI	Physiological Intracytoplasmic Sperm - A technique used in ICSI to find the healthiest sperm.

PID	Pelvic Inflammatory Disease - An infection spreads from the vagina to the cervix, the endometrium (lining of the uterus) and the fallopian tubes.
PIO	Progesterone in Oil Injection - This intramuscular injection is to thicken the uterine lining to protect the embryo and secure its healthy growth and development.
POAS	Pee On A Stick - Pregnancy test.
POF	Premature Ovarian Failure - Occurs when the ovaries stop functioning normally before age 40.
PUPO	Pregnant Until Proven Otherwise - An aphorism used in fertility groups, meaning that after an embryo transfer the woman will assume she is pregnant until a test tells her she is not.
RE	Reproductive Endocrinologist - Fertility specialist.
RO	Right Ovary
RPL	Recurrent Pregnancy Loss - Two or more pregnancy losses.
SA	Sperm/Semen Analysis - Assessment of the semen/sperm characteristics in the laboratory.
SC	Type of Injection - Subcutaneous, a short needle is used to inject a drug into the tissue layer between the skin and the muscle.
SD	Sperm Donor - A person who provides sperm for another person/couple to use.
Semen	Seminal fluid - Sperm containing fluid.
SI	Secondary Infertility - The inability to become pregnant or to carry a baby to term after previously giving birth.
SIUI	Stimulated IUI - Similar to IUI though given medications (FSH) to improve ovary response to produce a follicle.
Sperm Washing	Lab Procedure - Process where individual sperm are separated from the semen.
STD	Sexually Transmitted Disease - A condition passed from one person to another through sexual contact.
SURR	Surrogate - A woman who carries a pregnancy for another person/couple.
Surrogacy	Surrogacy - An agreement between a woman and another person/couple to carry a child for the parent/s.
TB	Testicular Biopsy - A procedure to extract sperm directly from the testicles.
TD	Treatment Day - Day of medical procedure.
TE	Trophectoderm - Blastocyst cells that form the placenta after implantation.
Teratozoospermia	Sperm condition - The presence of sperm with abnormal morphology.
TESA	Testicular Sperm Aspiration - Collection of sperm directly from the testis.
TESE	Testicular Sperm Extraction - Collection of from the tubules of the testis.
Testes/Testicle	Male Gonads - Male reproductive parts.
TL/TR	Tubal Ligation, Tubal Reversal - Sterilisation of the tubes, a permanent contraceptive solution.
Trigger	Injection - hCG injection given to induce ovulation.
TSH	Thyroid Stimulating Hormone - Produced by pituitary gland and stimulates the thyroid gland to release hormones.
TTC	Trying To Conceive - Attempting to have a baby.
TTCAR	Trying to Conceive After Reversal - Attempting to have a baby after a vasectomy reversal.
TWW	Two week wait - The waiting period between ovulation or fertility treatment and a pregnancy test.
Tx / Rx	Treatment - Medical care given to a patient.
US	Ultrasound / Sonography - Used to create imaging of fertility parts concerned.
Uterus	Womb - Site of the pregnancy.
V	Vasectomy - Male sterilisation by cutting the vas deferens to stop sperm reaching the ejaculate.
VR	Vasectomy Reversal - Reconnecting the vas deferens with view to allowing sperm to get to the ejaculate.

CONTRIBUTORS

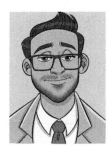

Dr Darren Katz is a Urologist and Male Fertility Microsurgeon who serves as Medical Director of Men's Health Melbourne – one of Australia's first integrated multidisciplinary clinics offering the latest approaches for the diagnosis, treatment and prevention of disorders affecting men's health and fertility.

A leading voice in male fertility treatment, Dr Katz is the Chairman and spokesperson of the Urological Society Australia and New Zealand Andrology Special Advisory Group. He is a Clinical Senior Lecturer at Melbourne University and a Director of the only Sexual Medicine, Male Infertility Microsurgery and Andrology Fellowship in Australia which attracts urologists from all over the world to train under his mentorship.

Dr Katz is heavily involved with research and academics and has been awarded both national and international grants and scholarships. He has been an invited faculty member for numerous urological workshops to teach other urologists and training urologists about the latest surgical techniques.

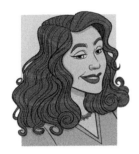

Dr Lynn Burmeister is the owner and Medical Director at No. 1 Fertility in Melbourne, Australia. She has worked in obstetrics and fertility for more than 20 years, and holds the highest degree for a fertility specialist called the CREI (Certificate of Reproductive Endocrinology and Infertility).

Dr Lynn completed this degree at the renowned Cornell University, studying and working with fertility leader Professor Zev Rosenwaks.

Her philosophy is simple: Dr Lynn's patients are "No. 1", and her clinics have the best and latest technology with state-of-the-art equipment and world leading scientists.

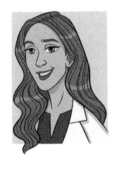

Dr Lora Shahine, MD, FACOG is a double board certified reproductive endocrinologist, Director of the Center of Recurrent Pregnancy Loss at Pacific NW Fertility, and Clinical Associate Professor in the department of obstetrics and gynaecology at the University of Washington in Seattle, WA, USA. Author of best selling *Not Broken: An Approachable Guide to Miscarriage and Recurrent Pregnancy Loss*, Host of *Baby or Bust* Podcast @drlorashahine on Instagram, YouTube, Tiktok, and most social media platforms.

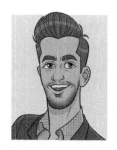

Dr Scott Shemer is an Obstetrician caring for women and their families in Melbourne, Australia. From normal to high-risk, Scott endeavours to provide dedicated, evidence-based, professional and compassionate care to pregnant women and couples throughout their entire pregnancy and birth. Scott's practice is located at Frances Perry House, the private wing of The Royal Women's Hospital. Scott has received awards for outstanding performance in the areas of obstetrics and gynaecology, paediatrics, medicine, surgery and psychiatry. www.drscottshemer.com.au

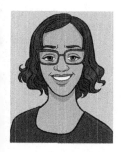

Sarah Jefford is a family creation lawyer, who helps families across Australia with surrogacy, donor conception and co-parenting arrangements. Sarah was an IVF mum, and later became an egg donor and a surrogate, giving birth to a baby in 2018 for two Dads. Sarah is the author of *More Than Just a Baby: A Guide to Surrogacy for Intended Parents and Surrogates.* Connect with her at www.sarahjefford.com

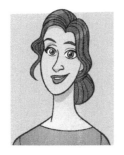

Tasha Jennings holds degrees in naturopathy, nutrition and herbal medicine and has more than 10 years of experience in the field. Continually inspired by innovative research, Tasha recently established her own company Zycia, which specializes in pre and postnatal nutrition to support life in its earliest stages. Follow Tasha @tashajenningsnd and download her Fertility Pantry checklist at https://tashajennings.com.au/checklistinfertilityman/

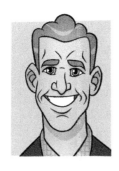

Dr Ryan Harrod chiropractor, is committed to chiropractic care, pro-active in his assessment, preventative management and empowerment of his patients. Graduating from the prestigious Royal Melbourne Institute of Technology Chiropractic double degree program, Dr Ryan has gained expert experience throughout Australia, working and volunteering his skills at various chiropractic clinics. Previously a professional sports person, Ryan has developed an intimate understanding of health, fitness and nutrition and continues to share this knowledge with his patients, and with other athletes.

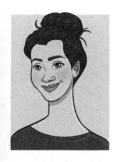

Tatiana Lawton is a freelance artist based in Sydney Australia. After graduating from Griffith Film School in Brisbane, Tatiana has worked on many Illustration projects; such as comics books, storyboarding for local films, and Illustrations for novels and children's books. She frequently has a table at Comic Con events around Australia promoting her latest artwork and projects. You can find her on Instagram at @tatianalarkinart or 'The Art of Tatiana L' on Facebook.

Made in the USA
Las Vegas, NV
18 November 2022